THE

METANOIA

PATH

CLAIM YOUR BEST ENERGY, HEALTH & HAPPINESS

Pam Frazier

Integrative Nutrition Health Coach

Disease Prevention and Reversal Guidance

Emmaus

Emmaus Wellness

ISBN 978-0-578-31845-5 | V05102024

EmmausWellness@gmail.com

UPDATED: May 2024

This book is dedicated to all the children in the world.
Together, let's lead them to the light of truth.

Contents

INTRODUCTION

Personal Wellness Journey

I choose what I become.

Life took a sudden directional change for Sharon, a favorite 60-year-old fitness student, when she suffered a stroke. Just after she went home from the hospital, her husband hired me as a personal trainer to help her regain balance and body movement. At our first session, I was not prepared to see Sharon lying on her bed with a tilted frown, an empty mood, and staring up to the ceiling.

"Hi, Sharon. How are you doing?" I asked when I walked in. Sharon was only able to grunt a response. My heart broke, and tears welled up in my eyes when I realized her speech ability was affected by the stroke. When I gently reached for her hands to check her sitting balance, she had no grasp and was unable to move. She then became a total weight lift as I pulled her up to a sitting position on the side of the bed. As I slowly released my hands from her shoulder and lower back, she immediately flopped back down to the bed, unable to sit for one second. This once vivacious and fun woman lived one month before her sad

1

departure from life.

Sharon's end of life was the first spiritual tap on my shoulder. It was time to leave the fitness profession and dust off my 21-year-old occupational therapy educational goals. Little did I know at that time that God had more plans for me. After serving thousands of patients in a 19-year medical career, being a Health Care Power of Attorney for three elderly female friends, and witnessing five dear friends transition from life one year, my knowledge and wisdom had increased about the human spirit, life, disease, death, and myself. These difficult experiences gifted me with blessings and a compassionate mark on my soul.

A second spiritual tap on my shoulder came as I witnessed my father succumb to heart disease, a highly preventable disease. I can remember him telling me, "Pam, aging ain't for sissies," as he struggled with his aging and disease process that included recovery from quadruple bypass surgery at the age of 71. After his surgery, he wondered out loud in my presence, "My dad died at 73, I wonder if I'll make it 'til then?" His dad had suffered a stroke at 58, and my father had his first heart attack at 52. Being the optimist he was, my father passed away two months after he turned 74. To this day, I believe that what we think, we attract to us. As you will read in this book, your attitude, lifestyle, stress levels, and all the choices you make are major factors in the balance of your energy, health, and happiness.

Not until my health was highjacked with rising blood pressure, cholesterol, glucose (all metabolic disorder precursors), and thyroid issues, did I know what it was like to be in the patient hot seat and filled with fear.

The third spiritual tap on my shoulder came after dealing with three physicians who did not offer me any HOPE, only cold-hearted prescriptions, a recommendation for thyroid surgery, and a lifetime of side effect-causing medications.

"How could this be happening to me?" I questioned. It felt like I faced a destiny of sickness with no chance of regaining my health and happiness. After an unethical and demeaning physician appointment, my mind was made up and I decided "NO WAY! is a sick destiny going to happen to me!" There was one problem, though. I didn't know where to start or whom to talk with for help. The only thing I knew to do was pray for help.

Then, on a cold December Sunday morning in 2013, Pastor Joy Nellissery's words woke up every ounce of my spirit as I sat in the church pew. His sermon, "Loving Our Holy Temple," made me feel as if I was the only one in church and his message was meant for me. As Pastor Joy closed his sermon, he stood firm and asked the congregation, "How are YOU treating your holy temple?" His question hit me between the eyes as I felt a shocking jolt throughout my body. My heart and mind were awakened like never before as I entered the Metanoia path, a spiritual path that would lead me to transform all my wrong choices. At that very moment, God's message told me to start treating myself like a newborn child in need of tender, loving care and to feed myself supreme nourishment in all areas of my life: body, mind, and spirit. God's light began shining on all the darkness in my life. I had been disconnected from God and had been suffering the consequences. My priorities and values were completely out of sync. Why was I ignoring God's will for my life and blocking His graceful blessings?

It was time to look at me in the mirror with an open mind and heart. The only person who could provide this tender, loving care was me, no one else. It was time to be accountable for my health, trust God, and accept His gifts of determination and perseverance to receive the healing He had planned for me ... and YOU.

Due to my Appalachian holistic genes, treating all my disease symptoms with pills and surgery was not the answer for me. The time had arrived to discover the causes of my health decline and learn how to reverse the ramping disease, my fear, and my imbalanced life.

I finally discovered the prescription no physician had ever written for me. This prescription included: mega doses of self-love, self-awareness, healing education, loving relationships, clean whole foods, water, quality sleep, joyful physical movement, life balance, faith, and HOPE. In a short amount of time, this prescription was filled. It was taken as directed: Daily, with the amount of needed dosage. Soon, my life was filled with unbelievable healing and joyful wellness. If this prescription worked wonders for me, it can work for you when you walk the Metanoia path by opening your mind and heart to God's will for your life. He wants the best for you!

Two weeks before this book went into its editing process, I asked God what He wanted me to use for the book title. As you read on the book cover and throughout this book, you see His answer: "Metanoia." When I saw Merriam-Webster's definition of Metanoia, it resonated with what was written in the book about opening your mind and heart to transform your body, mind, and spirit. "Metanoia" comes from the Greek word to change one's mind and repent. When we repent, we turn away from the things that are hurting us. When you embark on a wellness journey, as I did years ago, you will experience a change of mind about old habits. When you open your heart and mind to the light of truth, you will awaken like never before. This is when you step on the Metanoia Path, a spiritual walk that guides you to empowering choices to claim your best energy, health, and happiness.

Discovering the reasons disease enters our body, even our children's body is a major key. Being accountable for your health and the health of your children requires intentional and positive action to achieve a life of optimal wellness. The passion to write this book comes from a heart that served roles in the medical and healthcare profession as a therapist, patient advocate, fitness and wellness professional, and also as a daughter, a sister, a wife, a single mother, a grandmother, and most of all, a woman who has been saved by God's grace.

Today, I offer HOPE to you, your family, friends, and all the people in your life. Value your health as your true wealth in this life. Genuinely love your body, mind, and spirit as God loves YOU. You guide the quality of your life. When needed, start by forgiving yourself and others, then move into the present moment to receive the life you deserve.

May this book benefit you with self-accountability to walk your well-deserved Metanoia path.

CHAPTER 1

Awakened

The flower doesn't dream of the bee.
It blossoms and the bee comes. — Mark Nepo

This book was inspired early in my medical career as I served an elderly female patient who knew she had only a few days left to live. She had stopped eating except during our scheduled therapy sessions. Witnessing her acceptance of physical death taught me the gracious power of letting go as she journeyed to a new life.

Sharing 19 years of my life in the medical profession revealed to me that some patients were filled with hope, yet many others held blank stares of shock, confusion, fear, pain, sadness, tears, and denial about their health situation. All these diverse patients, their medical situations, and family members left a lasting imprint in my heart, my mind, and my emotional life. They required hospitalization and nursing care. Many received additional therapy, and some were recommended to hospice care.

The medical situations ranged from orthopedic problems, preventable to unpreventable diseases, and accidental injuries of all kinds. It was God who supported me when I met a patient whose hands were eaten away from a parasite tragedy and several patients who were in a tornado that damaged their health and home and had killed their loved ones. Before walking into many patient rooms, I would stand outside their door and pray for God's strength, words, and compassion to infuse my soul before our meeting. Witnessing patient sufferings could easily break my heart if it were not for God's strength and grace.

It is easy for medical professionals to become stressed by the multitude of their patients' emotions. Caring for patients during emergency urgent care, elective surgery care, and routine doctor office visits are all ways stress can be passed on to medical professionals when serving their patients. They are touched by all the choices their patients made in their life and also by the choices of others that crossed the patient's path. Choices made from the center of love spread love. When choices are made from conscious or unconscious self-centeredness, ignorance, neglect, denial, addiction, and hate, all of those vibrations radiate out to others who serve them.

Patients were presenting younger and younger in the last couple of years of my medical career. This evidence shows that our country is rapidly declining in family structure, values, and lifestyles. According to the Centers for Disease Control and Prevention (CDC), 42.4% of the U.S. population is obese, and childhood obesity is a serious problem. Obesity increases the risk for many serious diseases and health conditions.[1]

Heart disease, the #1 disease in the United States is highly preventable.[2] Obesity, Type 2 Diabetes, many cancers, and many other diseases are also preventable. These diseases are mainly created by a person's behavior, lifestyle choices, how they spend their time, and what they consume.[3] Unhealthy choices contribute to stress and an imbalanced lifestyle. If the stress and imbalance continue, disease begins to enter into the body, mind, and spirit. To put it in a nutshell, our country is being unconsciously guided by worldly temptations, which is a darkness many do not realize is destroying their health and happiness. Those who wake up and begin walking the Metanoia path of light can achieve optimal weight, health, and happiness.

Unbeknownst to many of us, a lot of our lifestyle patterns were set before we were conceived. Our parents' lifestyle, environment, and choice of food and drinks were all major influencers of our health and wellbeing. At the time of conception, our father's health was as much a major factor in our health as was our mothers'.

In a podcast, "How men's sperms can affect pregnancy," Dr. Kirtly Parker Jones, retired Vice-Chair of Education, Department of Obstetrics/Gynecology at University of Utah Health states: "Recent research has shown that genes encoded in men's sperm can be modified by the environment in which they were developing, and those modifications may affect the developing child." Once conceived, our mother's choice of food, drinks, habits, emotions, mental status, and lifestyle habits fuel our very own body, mind, and spirit as we develop in her body. Think about this: If you are addicted to a particular food, like sugar or salty foods, reflect on all the foods you were given as a child. Were you rewarded with certain foods when you complied with your parents' wishes? Did you get an apple or a sugar treat when you made good grades or made your parents happy and proud? What was stuffed in your Christmas stockings?

If you or someone you know want to have a child, please

share Dr. Kirtly Parker Jones's words: "We should tell men that are thinking of making a baby the same things we tell women. Clean up your act, eat well, maintain a healthy weight, try to manage your stress, and response to stress. Consider yourself an equal partner in the health of your future child, literally. It takes 90 days to make a sperm so let's get cracking, plan ahead, it'll be good for you."[4]

If your parents introduced you to any unhealthy food and drinks you crave today, please forgive them because they did not know what they were doing to you. Like most of us and many physicians, they did not know about the nutritional research facts we have at our fingertips today. The bottom line is: If you want better personal wellness, it is up to YOU to move beyond your past and into a brighter day and future.

PATIENT-PHYSICIAN RELATIONSHIP

Physicians are responsible for determining a patient's medical diagnosis and treatment. In non-emergency situations, you are the one who ultimately has the right to decide what happens to your body. Obtaining a living will and healthcare power of attorney is beneficial so your wishes will be honored if you become terminally ill, injured, or unconscious. Most of us employ a physician, and they in turn have the right to decide whether to accept us as a patient. A healthy relationship between a patient and physician involves mutual respect, trust, kindness, honesty, compassion, clear communication, and honor. Every United States physician is to follow standards set out by the Code of Medical Ethics of the American Medical Association (AMA).

I found it disheartening to witness patients and their family members in total confusion while in the hospital or a nursing rehab facility. Many did not know which way to turn when it was time to discharge home, nor did they realize their choices. Out of ignorance or fear, patients and family members failed to ask questions because they did not know what to ask.

Unfortunately, another occurrence I regularly witnessed was patients not receiving guidance or education. Upon discharge from a hospital or nursing rehab center they were only given cold direct orders from their physician or medical staff. There was no opportunity for the patient to ask questions or an opportunity for mutual discussion. This kind of situation involves an action of pride and power with no patient compassion or respect.

Patients have the right to pick and choose their primary physician, just like they do for any consumer service. Patients are customers who deserve compassionate care and respectful treatment at all times, no matter who is serving them. And, as a patient, your physician and their medical team deserve respect and clear communication from you regarding your concerns, questions, and goals.

Many times, I've heard disgruntled patients say, "No other physicians are accepting my insurance." This has never been the case during my 19 years in the medical profession. If you want to hire a new physician, word of mouth is your best resource. Ask your friends, family, co-workers, club members, and church members who they recommend. It's a good sign if you hear the same name several times. Your health insurance company may lead you in another direction, but know that it is ultimately your decision that will guide your medical service. Like all other businesses, physicians can accept or decline patients.

Physicians are not God and never will be. They are human beings just like you, me, and everyone else you know. They have challenges just like everyone else. What separates them from other business professionals is an earned medical degree and pledging an oath for the welfare of their patients. Typically, their income is derived from treating patients' symptoms by either prescribing medications, seeing their patients multiple times a year, ordering tests, providing surgery or other procedures, and possibly selling supplements or vitamins in their office.

How much time does your physician or his physician assistant or nurse practitioner typically spend with you? If you feel cheated in this area, ask your physician how many patients they see a day and how much time they typically spend with each patient. This will tell you a lot about your physician, their potential stress level, and how much personal face-to-face time their patients receive during an office visit. If you need more communication time with your physician or their team, ask for it.

One of my priorities as a new Integrative Nutrition Health Coach provider was to communicate my mission to all the physicians I served for many years. Many were verbally supportive, some were excited, and some looked bewildered, but comments made by two physicians saddened me. One, who had a private practice along with being a medical director, said, "Pam, people do not want to work at being healthy. All they want is to take a pill." The other physician said, "The spiritual component of a person's life has nothing to do with their health."

The person who reaches the top of the mountain with the help of a car or a train has not learned the lessons of the hiker on a wellness journey. To gain the beautiful vistas of health and happiness requires change in your lifestyle habits and daily choices. It takes daily determination and perseverance that no pill can offer.

Many physicians have a lot to learn about a person's ability to heal. Tremendous healing can happen when people are given

HOPE, proper education and resources, inspiration, support, time, and love.

Discussing your health goals with your physician and asking questions is essential for your wellness. Being accountable for your health shows that you value your wellness and quality of life. When you begin to share your goals with your physician, you may receive more support, guidance, and compassion.

To increase awareness about your physician-patient relationship, take a moment to answer these questions.

HOW'S YOUR RELATIONSHIP WITH YOUR PHYSICIAN?

- Are you comfortable asking questions during appointments with your physician?
- Does your physician exhibit respect when you ask questions or share comments?
- Does your physician offer patience and kindness during your time together?
- Does your physician offer a clear explanation of all prescribing tests or surgery recommendations?
- Does your physician review your labs and test results with you? Are you offered a copy of these results or access to an internet portal to access your records?
- Does your physician refer you to their business department to discuss the cost of all tests and surgery they order for you? Will your insurance pay for their recommended tests/surgery? How much money will you have to pay out of pocket?
- Are you offered information or resources to explain the benefits and side effects of all medications, tests, or surgery they prescribe?

- Does your physician offer you verbal education and referral resources to help you improve your health and wellness?
- Do you trust your physician?

WHICH PATIENT(S) ARE YOU?

- I'm an obedient patient and trust my physician 100%. I will do whatever I'm told.
- I'm a patient who asks questions and appreciates resource information and education so I can make wise decisions for the best health and quality of life.
- I'm a patient who complies with my physician only when I want to. Sometimes I don't and he/she may never know.
- I am a patient who does not comply with my physician's recommendations or orders.
- I'm a patient who will seek a second and third opinion when given a diagnosis or treatment I do not agree with.

Just like patients, physicians come in all shapes, sizes, and attitudes. Occasionally, a physician's diagnosis may be incorrect due to faulty lab results or your physician's incorrect assessment. When you are concerned about a diagnosis, consider seeking an additional opinion. No matter what a person's profession, human judgment may be driven by their emotions,[5] stress levels, mental and physical health, and lack of sleep. This is true for you and your physician. No one is perfect 100% of the time.

When you receive a diagnosis, it is your right to request

evidence and more information. If your physician does not want to comply, you may consider reaching out to another physician.

As an Integrative Nutrition Health Coach, an interesting discovery has come to me with each new client. Just like me during my sick past, many of my clients had imbalances in their life and nutrition. All were unaware of what caused their wellness declines. Hope for renewal never existed in their heart or mind because they never received any HOPE from their physicians. Witnessing all the hopeless patients in my medical career helped fuel the passion for my wellness journey, to become an Integrative Nutrition Health Coach, and to write this book.

Physicians who tell their patients the only answer to managing their health issue is by having surgery, radiation, countless chemo treatments, or a lifetime of medications are doing their patients a disservice. Physicians who open their minds and hearts to successful alternative methods for their patients to heal before ordering surgery or being exposed to toxic chemicals provide an avenue of hope and opportunity for the patient to reverse their damaging lifestyles.

Two major ways in which physicians can help support their patients in a non-emergency situation are to:

1. Offer patients immediate healing when they walk into your office by offering a calm and peaceful waiting room void of obnoxious TVs, commercials, and loud music. Allow them to feel peace and respect at all times when they are with you, your staff, and in your workspace. The benefits will be amazing for you and them.

2. Offer patients encouragement, inspiration, hope, guidance, and reliable resources to help them de-stress, create life balance, and improve their nutrition.

My hope is that physicians will learn what alternative and reliable resources are available to help patients learn to relax, balance their life, and eat healthily. These factors are essential for a quality life, optimal wellness, and disease prevention and reversal.

The medical maze confuses and frustrates people with its ever-changing research updates and the rising cost of insurance. As a patient, it is your right to know why you have been prescribed medications, tests, or surgery. If you want to live a life of health and happiness, make sure to kindly ask "Why?" every time you receive a new physician order or medication. If you wish to go an alternate route, ask if there is an alternative or noninvasive healing solution. If you are not in an urgent situation to commit to new medical orders, seek education to empower and inform yourself of any risks and symptoms caused by medications, supplements, procedures, and surgeries.

The internet has many educational avenues, so type in your question and you'll be amazed at the many resource links. New research and studies are going on every day in the science and medical field. What used to be a popular treatment five or 10 years ago may no longer be effective and may even cause harm to your body. Regarding medications, if you or someone you love happens to be 65 and above, the "American Geriatrics Organization Beers List" provides excellent guidance for unsafe medications and over-the-counter drugs. You will be amazed by the new recommendations about aspirin, other over-the-counter drugs, and medications prescribed by many doctors.[6] You can also review information about the BEERS list at *HealthAging.org*. Being a proactive consumer can protect your health, your quality of life, and save you precious time and money.

The key to knowing more is to seek and ask. Do not be afraid to ask questions or take time to research. It is your right to know as much as possible so you can make a wise and comfortable decision. Ultimately, it is up to you to be accountable for your health, the quality of your life, and your children's wellness. Ignorance, fear, and mindless habits will place your health and life in shambles if you allow it. Set yourself free and gain knowledge and wisdom.

When you are given a choice in life, do you think about the consequences for yourself and others? If not, begin incorporating three questions each time you make a choice or seek a new life direction.

1. Am I choosing a positive path?
2. Am I intentional with my thoughts and actions?
3. What will the circumstances be from my actions?

When all three of these questions are based on moral goodness, it's easier to achieve your goals, create positive lifelong habits, and love others. The best of intentions will fall apart when a person's actions and circumstances are misguided with worldly temptations. This will create hardship for the person who makes the misguided choices and for all who are involved in their life.

My purpose is to help you achieve the quality of life you desire. I want to help you envision it, create a plan, know how to take action, and let you know that you CAN get there by following your heart's desire when you walk the Metanoia path.

CHAPTER 2

Awareness:
The Foundation of Change

You find your power when you leave
your weaknesses behind.

If you want change in your life, you'll need to discover the roadblocks that may prevent success. Sometimes, God will place a barrier in your way to give you more time to listen to His guidance. So, it's essential to listen and follow peace and your heart's desire. Welcoming silence in your day will help open your mind and heart to what you desire in life.

LISTEN and SILENT are spelled with the same letters.

Wellness arrived in my life when I allowed more silence in my soul. This helped me become aware of my unconscious and poor choices, the creators of my imbalanced life. I was amazed to discover how worldly temptations and their deceptive ways had brainwashed me into the dark tunnels of disease. Discovering how to make wiser choices and why these choices were healing guided me out of this darkness as I climbed out to the light.

Thomas Merton's statement in his book, *No Man is an Island,* offers truth to achieving wellness: "Happiness is not a matter of intensity but of balance and order and rhythm and harmony."[1]

Achieving the life you desire begins with self-awareness. Learning about your body, mind, and spirit is essential to making wiser choices. Until you become aware of your daily choices and what drives them, you may blame your present wellness level on your destiny. Guess what? You hold the key to changing your life and the levels of your energy, health, and happiness.

Nourishing yourself with truth is the biggest step for positive growth and change. The truth will fuel your intentions and help focus your time on building a strong foundation.

LIFE BALANCE FOUNDATION

The **Life Balance Foundation** sample and tool, found on the following pages, was created to help you discover your present life balance. Once you complete the revealing **Life Balance Foundation** tool, it becomes the baseline for a wellness journey. The more you learn about the causes of your life imbalance, the better prepared you are to remove any roadblocks preventing the life you want.

Notice the 10 categories at the bottom of the **Life Balance Foundation** tool sample (next page). They are all essential for your overall wellness. On the left side are numbers ranging from 0 to 10, the life score ratings.

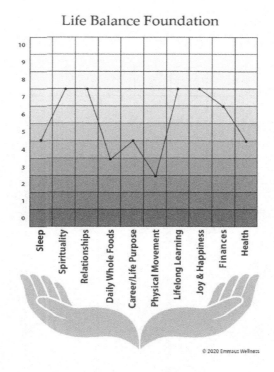

Life Balance Foundation

© 2020 Emmaus Wellness

To discover your life balance, complete the tool on the next page. Using a pencil or pen, place a dot on the number which best represents where you are for each category. The range is "0" (poor) to "10" (excellent).

Once you complete your 10 scores, connect the dots. The higher your category score, the more content you are in that area. Any low score creates an imbalance in your life, a roadblock to achieving what you want. Having balance in these five essential categories — sleep, spirituality, relationships, physical movement, and career or life purpose — offers you the strength to lift any low scores in the other five categories; daily whole foods, lifelong learning, finances, health, and joy and happiness.

Life Balance Foundation

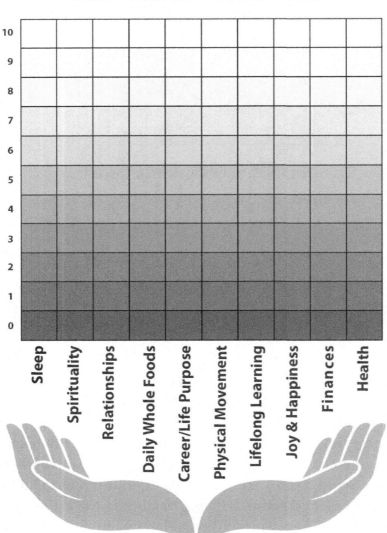

© 2020 Emmaus Wellness

Are you surprised by any of your **Life Balance Foundation** scores? Are there categories higher or lower than you expected?

Your scores can help you identify the choices and habits that cause cravings to tug at your brain when you least expect it. Our world is full of instant gratification, push buttons, and drive-thrus that divert your best intentions. This is what darkness does to us. It blinds us to the truth when we aren't aware of what's happening.

Unexpected life situations can also cause life imbalance, especially if you experience multiple happenings at the same time. Have you heard that life trials come in threes? I never believed it until my father's sudden death, my dear boss was suddenly fired, and a chaotic company takeover happened within a two-month timeframe. It didn't take long before my body started showing destructive signs from this combination of grief, stress, unconscious habits, and poor food choices. I'll never forget my physician asking me, "Pam what's going on in your life?" when he reviewed my yearly physical lab reports after these triple life adjustments.

Walking the Metanoia path creates balance in your life as you open your mind and heart to tenderly love yourself as God does. Accepting and implementing compassionate guidance and education from reliable resources are wise steps on this path. All of this helps to rewire your brain and calm the emotions of your heart. Your body will also go through a chemistry shift as healing takes place within you. This interior healing is the byproduct of realigning your perspective, beliefs, attitude, physical movement, and daily habits that release addictive cravings, emotional pain, loneliness, unconscious choices, and confusion.

As you walk a wellness journey, you can feel a decrease in stress and an increase in your peace, energy, health, and happiness. Learning about your 10 **Life Balance Foundation** categories will help reveal the cause of your imbalances and improve your self-accountability. You will also discover how important it is to create protective boundaries around your garden of life which you will read about in Chapter 12, "Setting Healthy Boundaries."

LIFE BALANCE CATEGORIES

SLEEP

Did you know one-third of your life is meant for healing sleep? The better your sleep patterns, the more your body can remove any built-up toxins in your brain and body tissues caused by mental, physical, or emotional debris from your day. Healing sleep positively affects all of your 12 body systems and 79 organs as you will learn in Chapter 6, "You Are A Miracle." Imagine healing rays traveling from your brain to your heart, lungs, and all your other 77 organs within your 12 body systems. These healing rays help boost your metabolism, immune function, mood, and disease resistance. If you experience chronic poor sleep, there is a breakdown of healing rays increasing the risk of many health disorders including high blood pressure, cardiovascular disease, diabetes, depression, and obesity.[2] In Chapter 13, "Healing Sleep," you'll find helpful guidance to improve your sleep.

SPIRITUALITY

How you nourish your heart and mind will make a difference in your daily peace and overall wellness. Spiritual nourishment increases your gratefulness, self-esteem, compassion for yourself and others, and improves relationships.

Spirituality can mean different things to different people. For some, participating in an organized religion creates their spiritual foundation. Other people may connect to a divine entity as a way to gain spiritual nourishment. Having faith and a spiritual practice can offer a better understanding of the mysteries of life and help one deal with the many worldly temptations and challenges. Some people meditate, some worship, some pray, and some go to nature to balance their hearts and minds. Some questions to ask yourself:

- Do I worry a lot?
- Is it hard to let go of people and things?
- Are my actions intentional, scattered, or impulsive?
- Am I driven by personal desires, or do I truly want to do for others as I would have them do unto me?

When beginning my wellness journey, writing down what I was most grateful for in a journal allowed me to express my heart, release my thoughts, and label my feelings with pen and paper. This practice continues to be a regular morning ritual that centers my entire being for the day. As I developed spiritually, more wellness entered my life. That's when I came to believe we are all spiritual beings in a physical form, and I allowed more time for silence and reading inspiring words of wisdom from the Bible and other spiritual books. Later on, I began including daily prayers for others that evolved into a prayer list. Now I ask God, "What can I do for you today?"

Starting the day feeling refreshed and blessed is so much better than being stressed.

RELATIONSHIPS

The most important relationship you have on this earth is the one between you and God, or your divine being. Relationships with your family, friends, mentors, and others, all contribute to your **Life Balance Foundation**. Positive relationships lift us, but negative ones pull us down. I was empowered when I learned how to obtain and maintain my self-respect. That was when I began setting protective boundaries with toxic patterns and negative relationships. Answer these questions and reflect on your present relationships:

- How is my self-respect level?
- How do my primary relationships affect my life?
- How do I get along with my parents, siblings, boss, co-workers, and all the other people in my life?
- If you have children, are they happy and content?
- How many younger people are in your life? (It's a plus to have all age groups in your life.)

If you find it difficult to set healthy boundaries in your life, Chapter 12, "Setting Healthy Boundaries," offers some helpful tips. My favorite Christian psychologists, Dr. Henry Cloud and Dr. John Townsend, have provided me with valuable lessons in personal respect, healing, and love via their books, websites, and Facebook sites.

DAILY WHOLE FOODS

Daily consumption of water, a variety of whole fruits, vegetables, whole grains, proteins, and healthy fats, instead of processed drinks and foods, will provide your body with the healthy nutrients it needs to energize, maintain, and enhance your overall health and wellness. This book will provide you guidance I've used to reverse disease in my body, mind, and spirit. Above all things, please remember that variety is the spice of nutrition. Be adventurous and creative with your drink and food choices to keep you from consuming the same thing over and over each day. Choosing a varied mix of daily nutritious choices in moderation will help you receive more empowering nutrients. In Chapter 8, "Your Food Choices Matter," be sure to read these sections: "Overdoing A Good Thing" and "Pay attention to Portion Sizes."

LIFE PURPOSE/CAREER

You have many natural-born gifts and talents, along with a divine plan for your life. Discovering and accepting your divine plan allows your natural gifts and talents to flow out to the world. In return, you will receive many blessings, for as you sow, you will reap.

Some may say their "calling in life" is also their life purpose. Volunteering or having a professional career that utilizes your many gifts and talents not only enhances your life but can also improve your wellness when balanced with your other **Life Balance Foundation** categories.

Think back to all the different stages in your life and where you are today. Time being one of your most valuable assets, how much time do you devote to your life purpose or career? Your answers to the following questions will provide you self-awareness.

- Do you feel at peace and content in the ways you share your time?
- Does your life purpose or career offer you time to care for yourself, your family and friends, your home, as well as time to enjoy your hobbies?
- Are there any changes you would like for your present life purpose or career?

PHYSICAL MOVEMENT

Regular physical movement provides many wellness benefits. When you participate in joyful daily movement, notice how your blood pressure lowers, your mood improves, and stress releases from your body, mind, and spirit. You also gain more energy, strength, flexibility, and happy hormones. On top of all of these benefits, physical movement helps deliver healing oxygen throughout your body and transports the nutrients from your food choices to your body's 12 systems and 79 organs via your internal blood flow.

As we reach the third decade in life, our muscle mass begins to decline a little each year. If you intentionally stay strong as you age, you will bypass the medical diagnosis of *sarcopenia* which I've encountered in reading many patient charts. Sarcopenia is a loss of muscle mass, muscle strength, and physical function. To combat sarcopenia, arm yourself with joyful physical movement, regular resistance exercise, and empowering nutrition.[3]

Staying strong is a top priority in my life, especially after reversing the onslaught of disease in my body and witnessing the regretful sadness in thousands of medical patients. If your physical movement had a low score on your **Life Balance Foundation** tool, make it a top priority in your life.

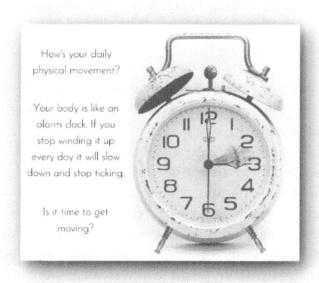

How's your daily physical movement?

Your body is like an alarm clock. If you stop winding it up every day it will slow down and stop ticking.

Is it time to get moving?

The more different types of movement you enjoy, the more fun it will be to stay strong. Dancing, hiking, biking, kayaking, working out with weights, pool time, yoga, walking around the neighborhood and the local greenways all bring joy to my life. Preparing your food, gardening, making your bed each morning, house cleaning, washing your car, and mowing your lawn are types of empowering physical movements.

Being strong is essential for wellness. Answer the questions below to discover what your present strength and physical movement levels are today.

- Do you have the energy and strength to do the things you consistently need to do in maintaining yourself and your home?
- How much time and how often are you physically active each day and week? Do you enjoy it?

- How is your balance while standing on your left foot for 10 seconds? How is your balance standing on your right foot?

Your body is your 24/7 home, and God created it to offer you a quality life. Being strong in your body also delivers vibrance to your mind and spirit.

The old saying, "If you don't use it, you lose it," is so true! During rehab patient discharge sessions, I would tell my patients, "This is our last therapy session before you go home. Please continue doing your therapy exercises at home. You will lose all the strength you gained within two weeks if you stop." Sadly, some of these patients returned to the rehab center because they did not maintain their positive physical movements from our therapy sessions. I hope you choose to avoid this pain in your life.

LIFELONG LEARNING

When the most important organ in your body, your brain, stays active, excited, and filled with new adventures, it too will be strong and vibrant. Remember when you were a kid and how you felt during those fun vacations and school time?

Traveling, learning to play a new instrument, meeting new people, trying out a new sport, and studying any subject that intrigues you are types of lifelong learning. The study, *The Impact of Sustained Engagement on Cognitive Function in Older Adults: The Synapse Project,* states: "Sustained engagement in cognitively demanding, novel activities enhance memory function in older adulthood. This research is clear evidence a person's memory function is improved by engagement in demanding everyday tasks."[4] Did you know the age of 60 is classified as the beginning of older adulthood from many health resources?

No matter what your age, what would you like to learn or do that you've never done before? If you carve out time for this desire, your action will decrease boredom and enhance your joy and happiness.

JOY AND HAPPINESS

Your emotional health is a vital part of your overall wellness. Negative thoughts and emotions can trigger an increase in stress hormones affecting your heart rhythm and nervous system that causes a decrease in your energy, daily performance, and mental clarity. A life filled with negative thinking and neglecting your divine being is similar to eating junk food every day. It will eventually rob your energy, health, and happiness.

Replacing negative thoughts and actions with positive ones will help renew your emotions. Releasing past hurts, forgiving others who caused you pain, and forgiving your neglect and self-harms are part of the renewal process.

Discover what fills your heart with joy and happiness and let it be in your life as much as possible. Simple nature pleasures like watching butterflies, listening to the songs of birds, watching ocean waves, and feeling the breeze on your body can fill your heart with joy and happiness. Sharing hugs with your loved ones, friends, family, and sweet pets also create beams of joy.

One joyful moment I'll never forget happened while eating lunch with my twin grandchildren when they were 34 months old. "Hey, Mason and Ava, what makes you happy?" I asked. Mason smiled big and shouted out "Food!" as he continued to eat homemade lasagna. "Helping people," Ava softly answered. As Mason continued to eat, he humbly chimed in again and said "Sharing." How is it possible these young children were able to respond with simple truths of joy and happiness? As a family, they hold hands with their parents before each meal and say out loud: "We are family and we do awesome things. We love each other, we are thankful, we are helpers. We are patient and kind." The foundation parents create for their children influences their thoughts, actions, compassion for others, and self-esteem. This daily family ritual affects Mason and Ava's hearts and connects with their brain, creating their positive thinking pattern.

During our life journey, we meet people who teach us valuable lessons about life and ourselves. One of my favorite poems says it all:

"People come into your life for a reason, a season, or a lifetime. When you figure out which it is, you know exactly what to do.

When someone is in your life for a REASON, it is usually to meet a need you have expressed outwardly or inwardly. They have come to assist you through a difficulty, to provide you with guidance and support, to aid you physically, emotionally, or spiritually. They may seem like a godsend, and they are. They are there for the reason you need them to be.

Then, without any wrongdoing on your part or at an inconvenient time, this person will say or do something to bring the relationship to an end. Sometimes they die. Sometimes they walk away. Sometimes they act up or out and force you to take a stand. What we must realize is that our need has been met, our desire fulfilled; their work is done. The prayer you sent up has been answered and it is now time to move on.

When people come into your life for a SEASON, it is because your turn has come to share, grow, or learn. They may bring you an experience of peace or make you laugh. They may teach you something you have never done. They usually give you an unbelievable amount of joy. Believe it! It is real! But, only for a season.

LIFETIME relationships teach you lifetime lessons; those things you must build upon to have a solid emotional foundation. Your job is to accept the lesson, love the person/people (anyway); and put what you have learned to use in all other relationships and areas of your life. It is said that love is blind but friendship is clairvoyant."

— *author Unknown*

Many of us believe we can be happy when we have someone or something that brings instant pleasure into our lives. The problem with this concept is that no person or any material possession can bring you the gifts of joy and happiness because it's an internal process within your divine being.

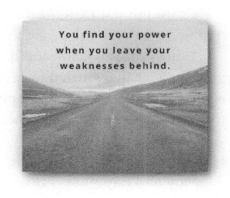

You find your power when you leave your weaknesses behind.

Pleasure is a sensation and biochemical response that comes to us from the external world. Pleasures are not part of our inner being. They are typically found in a bowl of ice cream, money, power, buying something new, gambling, drinking alcohol, taking drugs, or something erotic that pulls us away from the light of truth. All of these pleasures create unbelievable chemical changes within our body and brain. They easily misguide our best intentions and can steal joy and happiness from the depths of our hearts.

Obtaining self-awareness will help you discover your true essence and your inner truth, a path to joy and happiness. This discovery helps you build the courage to leave weaknesses that have blocked your life balance and overall wellness.

Accepting your internal gifts and learning what brings you real joy and contentment increases self-love and respect. This will lead you to live your true purpose and realize that simple things in life can bring you happiness and joy.

Happiness is a byproduct of your thoughts, intentions, and actions. It's not where you live that matters but how you live each day. A key to happiness is to intentionally maximize joy in your life and minimize stress, worry, anxiety, and poor choices.

For me, the joy of loving and honoring God, compassion for others, or sharing a sunrise kayak paddle with people who love to feel this adventure are examples of deep contentment. Holding hands with my grandchildren or being with a dear friend as we walk through nature's magnificent glory always brings joy and happiness to my soul.

What brings you joy and happiness? Take a moment to write your answer in a journal or on a piece of paper. Reflect on your answer. Are your joy and happiness levels where you want them to be? If not, what needs to change in your life to get there?

The more you surround yourself with situations that create blooms within your heart, the better your energy and health. True joy and happiness are awakened by a calm acceptance and appreciation of what you have and where you are in your present life, the foundation of a grateful mind, body, and spirit.

FINANCES

When you earn money to support your basic needs and can share it with others, you have reached a balance in your finances. Dave Ramsey, a leading financial guru, has said: "The thing I have discovered about working with personal finance is that the good news is that it is not rocket science. Personal finance is about 80 percent behavior. It is only about 20 percent head knowledge."

Financial wellness is a part of life balance, and, according to a person's choices, it may offer feelings of comfort, security, peace, or, on the other hand, a lot of stress. How is your financial peace today? If you need guidance, research on the internet to locate a *Financial Peace* class in your area or research the Dave Ramsey website: **https://www.ramseysolutions.com/**.

HEALTH

How is your score for your present health? Does your health enable you to do everything you want to do in life today?

As the ancient Roman poet, Virgil, wrote: "Health is your greatest wealth." When I placed my health as a life priority, amazing blessings came my way. Optimal wellness will provide abundant blessings of freedom and peace. My wish is to exit this physical life while laughing, not lying in a nursing home bed.

WHAT TO DO ABOUT THOSE LOW SCORES

At the start of my wellness journey, I was shocked by my first life balance scores. My "Joy and Happiness," plus a couple of major foundation categories, were very low. Reflecting on the causes for these low scores helped me identify roadblocks to having wellness in my life. It also pointed out that some of my stress was self-induced and some came from unexpected life happenings. The depth of my selfish goals, poor choices, distorted perceptions, mindless habits, and frustrations were major roadblocks. All these factors, mixed with ignorance and fear, created the developing disease in my body. I discovered that the most nutritious foods could never satisfy all my hunger for the best energy, health, and happiness, although nutritious food is an essential ingredient for gaining and maintaining wellness.

Your **Life Balance Foundation** scores provide a platform to set goals and to create a plan of action for the life you truly desire. Revisiting your **Life Balance Foundation** in one month, in three months, six months, and a year will help you see the progress from your first scores. Each time you retake your **Life Balance Foundation**, document the date so you can focus on your progress, your actions, and the amount of time it took you to achieve your goals.

An important part of accomplishing my wellness goals was forgiving all my past thoughts, actions, and poor choices. True forgiveness opened my heart and mind to all the blessings in my life, created daily gratefulness, and more peace entered my days as I began living in the present moment.

CHAPTER 3

Change:
A Constant in Life

The secret of change is to focus all of your energy not on fighting the old, but on building the new. — Socrates

Change is constant in our world. Humans, all living creatures, and nature adapt to daily change and may not notice when it happens. Just as the sun rises every morning, the sun will set each evening. As our body flows with the daily rhythm of change, we may ignore the significance of every hour unless an awesome memory was created or something difficult happened.

Many life changes can affect your balance within your physical, emotional, mental, and spiritual health. Think about these examples and how it has or would affect you: Sudden weather changes; beginning a new job or losing one; hearing a new medical diagnosis or experiencing a miracle healing; getting married or battling through a divorce; the birth of a child; school graduation; or experiencing the death of a loved one. Even though some of these changes are exciting to your heart and some are sad, they all can be difficult to accept and adjust to.

When it comes to personal change, nourishing your mind, body, and spirit is important. To achieve what you want, enter the Metanoia path by readjusting your mindset, opening your heart, and creating intentional behavior. The more realistic your goals, the more you will achieve them. The most successful clients I've met created obtainable goals from day one and stayed away from unreachable dreams they wanted immediately. This is a central step to achieving what you want in life.

To begin the desired change in your life, write down three goals you plan to act on and a definite date to achieve them. This will help you focus. If you don't meet your goals by your desired date, reset the date and get refocused to achieve the remainder of your goals.

Deep commitment activates your determination and perseverance. This will influence your daily intentions and bring more positive results. Along with a deep desire for change, obtaining new knowledge will open your mindset and help you understand why your old habits and choices created harm. In addition to reading many wellness and self-help books, attending the Institute of Integrative Nutrition empowered me with the knowledge to change my imbalanced life and poor habits. My wish is for you to receive these same blessings from reading and utilizing this book throughout your life.

Practicing a new habit every second, minute, and hour of each day will rewire your brain by creating new synaptic avenues. This process is called neuroplasticity. As it has worked for me, it will help rid you of damaging cravings and habits by replacing them with healthier choices and actions.

When I began to infuse my body with nutritious foods, my taste buds and biochemistry changed. As you introduce clean whole foods and water into your daily life, in time, your body will experience fewer cravings for highly processed sweets and sodium-induced foods and drinks. The daily infusion of high nutrient whole foods, water, and balancing my life helped to heal me. It can create healing for you too. The key is to be diligent, patient, and trusting.

When you become mindful of your thoughts and actions, this will introduce more peace into your day. Below are a few questions to reflect on when you wake up each morning. This morning ritual can offer you soul-centering that will open your self awareness, provide you answers, and guide you to better choices.

- How is my peace?
- What is my energy level?
- If my energy is low, what are the causes? What did I eat, drink, swallow, and place on my body in the last 24-48 hours?
- How is my stress level?
- What caused any stress I am feeling?
- Are low energy and stress caused by something I want or need in my life?
- Will these causes offer my life true value?
- How is my faith today?
- How is my patience today?
- Am I living in the moment, the past, or the future? Living in the past may create depression. Living in the future may create anxiety.
- My God, my divine power, what is your will for me today?

The answers to these questions will open doors to your past mindset and help you become aware of any doors that are still locked. If your peace and energy are low, reflect on these questions and, if needed, write your answers in a journal to help you release their hold on you.

As the sun rises and the moon sets, change enters our lives every day. When we learn how to invite peace into our day this helps us balance as the world turns.

CHAPTER 4

Understand Epigenetics

Create the change you want.

Gaining knowledge about epigenetics provided me more hope and determination to reverse the growing disease in my body as I began my wellness journey.

    "Epigenetics is the study of changes in gene function that are heritable and that are not attributed to alterations of the DNA sequence," states Laura Elnitski, Ph.D. of The National Human Genome Research Institute.[1] While there are no direct changes to our DNA sequence, one's lifestyle choices can turn their genes "on" or "off," making them respond positively or negatively. For example, the 30 trillion cells in my body responded negatively when I led an unhealthy lifestyle. When I started balancing my lifestyle, improving my daily nutrition choices, and decreasing my stress level, the disease process disappeared. The healing within my body, mind, and spirit verified how intentional and wise lifestyle choices reversed disease and prevented the history of family disease from impacting my life.

When your daily choices come from the center of love and are grounded with knowledge and wisdom, you'll receive more gifts of wellness. If your choices are unconscious and driven by worldly temptations, cravings can easily turn into addiction causing stress, pain, and unrest throughout your body, mind, and spirit.

If you truly want to change, intentionally take control of your life. Focus on loving YOU in every single way from the moment you wake up every day until you lay your head on the pillow at night.

The Danish Twin study[2] revealed that genetic differences account for about 20% of the variance in adult human lifespan, and 80% of non-genetic factors, such as lifestyle, dictate a person's longevity. To uncover the secrets of longevity, Dan Buettner, author of Blue *Zones*, teamed up with National Geographic, National Institute of Aging, demographers, scientists, and anthropologists and set off around the world to discover the secrets of living a long and fruitful life.

They discovered five different world locations, called the Blue Zones, where people consistently live more than 100 years. This age group is known as centenarians reside in these locations:

1. Loma Linda, California, USA
2. Sardinia. Italy
3. Okinawa, Japan
4. Nicoya, Costa Rica
5. Ikaria, Greece

Nine evidenced-based denominators were discovered among the centenarians in each of the Blue Zones. They are now called the Power 9.

THE POWER 9

1. Their home environments require daily physical movement to maintain their home, gardens, and property without mechanical conveniences.
2. They consumed light evening meals and only filled up to 80% capacity during all meals.
3. Most meals were plant-based using beans, soy, and lentils for protein. Very little meat was eaten except for a small, 3-4 ounce serving of pork being consumed approximately five times per month.
4. Little to no alcohol was consumed. When it was, it was shared with friends or during a meal.
5. They wake up each day with a known purpose, sharing their time and talents with others.
6. Their stress-reducing habits included gratefulness, prayer, naps, and happy hour.
7. Most gathered with a faith-based community each week.
8. Family is their top priority relationship.
9. They have strong social networks with supportive healthy values.

As you can see, the Blue Zone centenarians have many years of health and joyful balance in their lives. Other family studies reveal healthy aging and longevity in humans is about 25% due to genetic factors. This proves the power of a healthy lifestyle supersedes the theory that diseases are caused by 100% genetic factors, as many physicians promote.[3] Before my wellness journey began, a former physician encouraged me to take blood pressure medication to prevent a stroke or heart attack like my father and grandfather experienced in their lives, even though my blood pressure was not regularly high. An episode of job strain or emotional stress can easily affect a person's normal blood pressure as it had done to me. It's chronic stress that can keep one's blood pressure high.

Much of today's diseases are caused by a person's daily choices. Below are proven primary choices that damage human health. Are any of these choices part of your life today?

- Regular consumption of processed food and drinks
- Drinking too much soda, caffeine, and alcohol
- Little to no daily physical movement
- Allowing stress to rule your body, mind, and spirit
- Toxic relationships
- Little to no spiritual life
- Stress, loneliness, unbalanced life, and emotional struggles

Several of these choices were part of my daily life during my past health decline phase, especially the stress, poor food and drink choices, toxic relationships, and an imbalanced life. Understanding the importance of your lifestyle choices and how they contribute to your health or cause disease is important.

Are you becoming more aware of what may cause discomforts in your life? The beginning of wellness is to understand when and how those choices began in your life. After you discover those answers, your next step is to open your mind and access more education to gain what you want in life.

Once you discover how any unhealthy habits were formed, forgiving all the situations that led to your choices will give you freedom, especially if you've been holding on to hurt. With the gift of freedom, renewal and peace will come into your heart and mind.

Understand this: YOU hold the epigenetic key to turning on or off your wellness depending on your daily choices. The more you learn, the more you will understand, and the more YOU CAN improve your quality of life.

CHAPTER 5

Beginning A Wellness Journey

I am claiming my life.
It springs forth with intention and self-love.

The most important question to ask yourself when you want change in your life is: What do I want?

Time is your most valuable asset and pursuing what you want must become a daily priority. As Harvey Mackay, a successful author and businessman stated: "Time is free, but it is priceless. You can't own it, but you can use it. You can't keep it, but you can spend it. Once you've lost it, you can never get it back."[1]

Take time now and complete the **Time Wheel** on the next page to see how you spend your time on an average day.

To begin, first block out your daily sleep and personal self-care times. Next, block out the average time you spend on your career or life purpose, driving, home maintenance, cooking, meal times, rest or nap times, shopping, family and friendship time, community and church time, internet, TV, social media, etc. The more specific you are, the more you will see how you spend your time.

THE TIME WHEEL

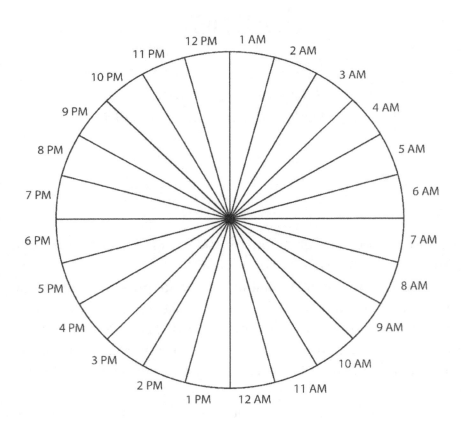

ASK YOURSELF THESE QUESTIONS:

- Am I spending time on my life priorities?
- Am I spending time on what I value?
- What activities delete time from my goals?
- How much free time do I have each day?

DAILY TIME LOGS

To increase your self-awareness about how you spend your daily and weekly time, keep a written log for one to two weeks. Keeping track of what you do and how much time you spend on each activity will help you uncover unconscious patterns. When you see the facts, you can better prioritize your time according to what you want in life.

UNCOVER YOUR PATTERNS

When you see where you are spending your time, you will see what is preventing you from achieving your goals. Reducing or removing life-draining habits and time wasters is essential. Plan to replace any time wasters with positive action to reach your goals.

GET ORGANIZED TO PRIORITIZE

To reach your goals, decide what needs to be done daily and weekly. Review your **Life Balance Foundation** scores and focus on balancing any of these six main categories if they are low: Sleep, relationships, whole foods, spirituality, career or life purpose, and physical movement. Allowing daily time to improve these areas is essential for your overall wellness.

COMMUNICATE YOUR GOALS

Sharing your goals with those closest to you will reveal who will support and respect you during your wellness journey. Being sabotaged by a close relationship who creates the temptations you are trying to avoid will make your journey difficult. Surround yourself with supportive and healthy relationships to help you achieve your goals, and ask for support when you need it.

WHAT IF I GET SIDETRACKED?

Confucius has a perfect message for everyone walking a wellness journey: "Our greatest glory is not never falling, but in rising every time you fall." When you fall away from your goals reflect on these questions:

- What are my goals?
- How is my focus?
- Am I setting clear deadlines?
- Are my days organized or chaotic?
- Do I allow wasteful interruptions? If so, name them.
- What choices are getting me closer to my goals?
- Do I allow time to relax in my day?
- Do I have a grateful attitude?

As I have noticed in my life and you may notice in yours, too much structure can take the joy out of living, and too much available time can create boredom. Balancing your time will get easier as you release wasteful habits and bring in productive actions. When you get sidetracked, review your goals and review or retake your **Life Balance Foundation** tool.

Taking an honest look in the mirror helps one to see their internal reflection. For me, it was like turning on a bright light in a dark room. The light uncovered my thoughts and behavior that blocked peace, self-love, hope, and life balance from being in my life.

During our day, we all face worldly temptations that divert us from being soul-centered. Most diversions are rooted in pride, envy, anger, laziness, greed, gluttony, and lust. Make time to think about your internal reflection. It will help you identify the source of negative habits, perceptions, attitudes, and patterns that are preventing you from getting what you want in life.

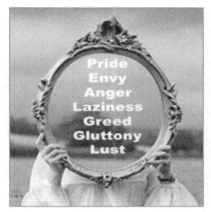

FACTS TO REMEMBER

- Unexpected events will occur in life. You may need to bend at times.
- Temptations are everywhere! You CAN conquer them.
- Uncontrollable cravings can have a tight hold on you. Tackle your worst craving first.
- Mindless time zappers can easily control your brain's focus. Kiss them goodbye!
- If you fall off track, forgive yourself, dust yourself off, and get back on track. Always remember: YOU deserve the best life!

Your wellness journey begins by opening your mind and your heart to three very important lifetime commitments:

1. Self-respect
2. Self-love
3. Patience

To achieve what you want, you must envision the life you desire. Believe you deserve the blessings, take daily action, and fuel yourself with determination and perseverance. That space between your vision and reality is measured by your daily determination and perseverance.

WRITE IT DOWN

As mentioned in Chapter 3, "Change – A Constant in Life," setting realistic goals and committing to a definite date will help you stay focused on achieving your goals. In Chapter 16, "Get SMART, Get Ready Go!" you receive guidance to fine tune your goals. For example, if you desire to increase your physical movement each week, state how many days per week, what type of movement, and how much time you plan to reserve for this new goal. Just like any other important appointment, create time for joyful physical movement on your daily calendar to prevent wasteful habits from robbing your commitment.

The best goal reminder for me is writing my top three goals on a sticky note and placing the sticky note on my bathroom mirror. Other places to post your goals could be on your refrigerator, pantry door, car dashboard, or computer screen. Placing your goals on your cell phone display, or in its calendar, is another good place. You will see these reminders multiple times a day and that will help your brain focus on doing new habits to achieve your goals.

When I made up my mind to create changes in my health and professional life, writing in a journal became a true gift. The writing pattern was sporadic at first, yet in time it became a daily morning practice to release my thoughts, feelings, and to lift gratitude from the depths of my being. It now creates an avenue for clarifying my path and opens my mind to listen and follow divine guidance. When I finish journaling, I read parts of three daily inspirational books, the Bible, and other divine wisdom to fill my soul with spiritual nutrition. This practice fuels me with daily peace, a protective shield to worldly temptations. The three daily inspirational books, which all came to me as gifts, are *My Utmost For His Highest* by Oswald Chambers, *God Calling* by A.J. Russell, and *Jesus Calling* by Sarah Young.

Are you ready to start a wellness journey today? If so, one of the best things you can do is to write down your questions and answer them in a journal. A simple spiral notebook or your computer can be used. Journaling helps when you are at a crossroads in life and not sure which direction to go. Writing down questions and answers in a journal also provides remarkable guidance. You'll be enlightened when you read your personal growth and accomplishments once you review your past journal entries from a month, three months, and up to a year. Below are some questions from my earliest journals you may wish to use:

- What is missing in my life?
- What do I want in my life?
- What are my time zappers?
- Dear God, what should I do?

Another important question to ask yourself: What do I **_not_** want in my life? Answering this question will help reveal barriers to what you want in life. You may already know how each barrier makes you feel, although writing it down will begin your release process. For each barrier answer these questions:

- Does this offer value to my life?
- Does this offer me energy or deplete my energy?
- Does it take time away from my priorities?
- What can I do to remove the barrier?

Removing a barrier may take time. It may require personal acceptance for each one and a change in your perceptions. Some major barriers that prevented my wellness journey were toxic relationships, fear of leaving a lucrative professional salary, and lack of faith. If you have more than three barriers, work on the three easiest ones first. When you've successfully removed them from your life, work on more until they are all gone. Preparation, education, hope, prayer, and renewed faith were the most helpful gifts in removing these barriers from my life.

One month before leaving the medical profession, I woke up at the usual time and sat up on the side of my bed. As my feet touched the floor, I heard a voice whisper, "Do not be afraid." That was the moment when I knew it was time to make the career move I had feared for two years. The time had arrived for my new life purpose to educate, inspire, and guide others to claim their best energy, health, and happiness. This spiritual experience happened right after I had dissolved all barriers blocking what I wanted in life. Divine timing is truly perfect.

If you fear that other people will read your journal, this can be easily solved. Write or type whatever you desire to express, receive your well-deserved release, and, when ready, release your words in a spiritual method I've used for many years. This practice is called the Burn Jar.

This small 5" x 6" Burn Jar is what I use to release written words I prefer to remain secret between God and me. With my written words in hand, along with the Burn Jar and a lighter, I walk outside onto my patio where there is no danger of starting an uncontrolled fire. Once the paper is crumbled inside the Burn Jar, I touch a

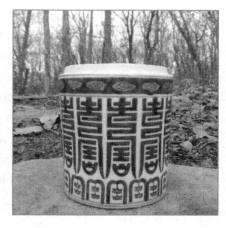

corner of the paper with a flame from the lighter. As my written words begin to burn and the smoke rises, I pray to God to accept the situation that was in my heart and mind. Watching the paper completely burn helped to release any unhealthy attachments I may have been experiencing and needed to release. To finalize the Burn Jar process, I wet the ashes and place them in the dirt for a complete grounding release.

In addition to journaling, some people use meditation, also known as mental prayer, to help them focus on their goals. It is a very simple process involving your mind and heart focus. Prayer, communicating with a divine being, is another way people seek guidance and strength. Prayer and listening to God's guidance provide me daily peace. Prayer is especially helpful when I want to support other people or I am dealing with a new crossroad or a worldly temptation that entered my path. As it has been for me, divine guidance arrives at the right time. Sometimes answers can come in the form of a whisper, in a dream, written words, or spoken words from a known person or a stranger. Divine answers also come in one of three messages: "Yes," "No," or

"Wait." A lot of hardship can be avoided in your life if you accept and obey the given answer along with being patient, especially if you receive the "Wait" guidance.

YOU are the only one who can remove the barriers to having what you want in life. If you have fear, do not be afraid to reach out for help. Reach out to a wise friend, a trusted family member, a professional mentor, a church leader, or a recommended counselor. You can even reach out to me.

Looking back at the inspiration for my present life purpose, God was tapping me on the shoulder to straighten out my life imbalances and poor habits. He knew there was no way I could help others until I walked the Metanoia path to claim my best energy, health, and happiness.

Yes, you will be doing a lot of new things. Your vision of a new life can spring forth with your best intentions and self-love. When you sincerely desire a new life, think it, act on it, and claim it! Be diligently patient and persevere every day. Believe YOU are a miracle and worthy of supreme love!

CHAPTER 6

You Are A Miracle!

*Take a look inside; you will be amazed
at your miraculous design.*

Amazing benefits come your way when you gain knowledge about your body, its functions, and all the interconnections. Achieving your best wellness is an inside-out job, so learn as much as you can about YOU and YOUR 24/7 home.

When you realize your body is your personal 24/7 home, it's easier to understand why it requires ongoing maintenance for a quality life. Similar to most engines, to run at peak performance, your body needs proper fuel, active and rest time, occasional balancing, tune-ups, and regular cleaning to look and feel great during your life journey.

Maintaining your 24/7 home with positive choices provides the best life balance, peace, and vibrance. Think of this book as an owner's manual to care for your unique miracle.

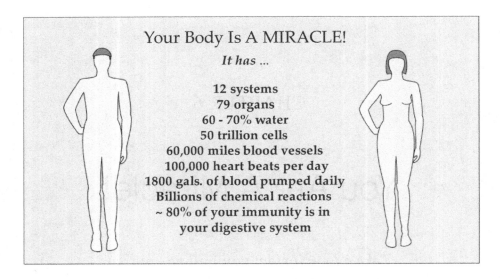

Your Body Is A MIRACLE!
It has ...

12 systems
79 organs
60 - 70% water
50 trillion cells
60,000 miles blood vessels
100,000 heart beats per day
1800 gals. of blood pumped daily
Billions of chemical reactions
~ 80% of your immunity is in
your digestive system

THE IMPORTANCE OF HYDRATION

First and foremost, for humans to even exist, we must receive daily and adequate hydration. We can only live about three days without it because our entire body is approximately 60-70% water. On the following page, take a look at a couple of your vital body parts and see how much water is in each one.[1]

Amazing, isn't it? Water is everywhere in your body! Drinking water, not soda drinks or energy drinks, is essential for peak performance. Below are some important roles water provides you:

- Creates saliva for your digestion process.
- Helps lubricate your joints.
- Helps your kidneys eliminate toxins and waste products from your blood and urine, and processes water-soluble toxins from your liver.

- Helps convert food into components for digestion assistance.
- Helps create brain hormones and neurotransmitters.
- Acts as a shock absorber for your brain and spinal cord.
- Helps deliver oxygen throughout your body.
- Helps regulate your body temperature via sweating and respiration.

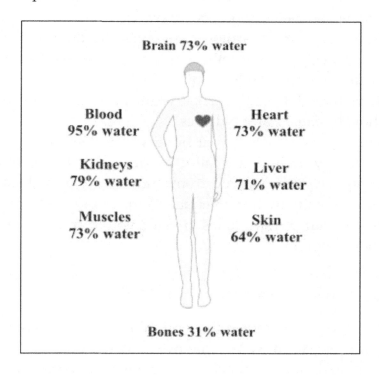

If your body is low on water, a condition called dehydration can occur. Some of the symptoms include fatigue, dizziness, confusion, headaches, constipation, hunger, muscle cramps, dry mouth, feeling overheated, and your skin not bouncing back after a light pinch. If you have one of these symptoms it would be wise to keep track of your daily water intake, observe how you feel each day, and make water consumption adjustments as needed.

DAILY HYDRATION TIPS

Depending on your present health, physical activity levels, the weather, and your surrounding environment, your water needs may be different than others. The U.S. Geological Survey (USGS), the sole science agency for the Department of the Interior, states: "An adult male needs about 3 liters (3.2 quarts) per day while an adult female needs about 2.2 liters (2.3 quarts) per day. All the water a person needs does not have to come from drinking liquids, as some of this water is contained in the food we eat." Many fruits, vegetables, broth, soups, and yogurt contain water. Some fruits and vegetables containing large amounts of water include watermelon, strawberries, pears, peaches, lettuce, celery, Bok Choy, tomatoes, and radishes.

Many times, you may feel hungry when in actuality your body is thirsty. Drinking a tall glass of water may relax those hunger signals and save you from unnecessary added calories. Discover the daily hydration equation that makes you feel your best unless your physician has directed you to abide by another hydration program.

CAUTION: TOO MUCH HYDRATION CAN HARM YOU

Sometimes we think more of a good thing can help us reach our goals quicker. When we become overzealous and do more than recommended, this can backfire. After a wellness presentation, a gentleman approached me and said he had tried to lose weight by drinking a lot of water. Unfortunately, he was admitted to the hospital and was diagnosed with hyponatremia. His excess water intake caused his body's sodium levels to drop to a near-fatal level that affected his body cells and created a lot of swelling. Luckily, it did not harm his brain as has happened to many people after consuming too much water.

WHAT TOUCHES YOU AFFECTS YOU

Everything you put into your mouth, swallow, inhale, and place on your skin is broken down inside your body. It is then transported throughout your body via your blood. Your body has 60,000 miles of blood vessels that travel to the tips of your fingers, your heart, your toes, all over, around, up, and down your entire body including your most important organ, your brain.

We are constantly bombarded with visual marketing enticement by the processed food and restaurant industries to increase product sales so the owners and stockholders will make money. Many companies intentionally use addictive ingredients, including sugar, sodium, and caffeine to create their products. So, BEWARE of all the marketing hype constantly around you. It is cleverly created to tempt and hook everyone, including you, and our innocent children.

Our constant cravings for addictive food and drinks can lead us to unconscious habits and higher consumption levels. These processed products trigger the pleasure center in our brain causing imbalances in our body's chemistry that also affect our mood and mental state. This happens as the opiate receptors get stimulated in our brain by one, some, or all of our five senses: taste, sight, smell, touch, and hearing. Dopamine, also known as the "happy hormone," is then released from our brain creating pleasingly high moods and warm fuzzies throughout our entire body. The more pleasant our highs, the more we crave. In time, our health shield may weaken, allowing our family disease history to creep into our body. For example, my family disease history includes heart disease, diabetes, and thyroid disorders.

With all my past unhealthy food choices and poor lifestyle habits, my family diseases began showing up in my body. After initiating a wellness journey, these budding family diseases reversed and my body began to heal. Within months, my medical lab reports improved and all the physician-ordered prescriptions were deleted from my life.

Uncontrollable food and drink cravings are not the only challenges we humans suffer. Becoming mindful of all worldly temptations is important. Take notice if you feel you are experiencing laziness, gluttony, pride, lust, envy, anger, or greed in your body, mind, or spirit. If this happens, know that the distance between what you want and reality is measured by your discipline and perseverance.

Balancing every ounce of your body, mind, and spirit is essential to combat and defeat the worldly temptations that can blind you. As you make healthier lifestyle choices and consume more clean, whole foods, it will become easier to see the deceptive marketing traps that previously captured and held your brain hostage. Temptations are everywhere, and the more you distance yourself from them, the easier it will be to conquer them.

PILLS AND MORE

We are all unique individuals and what may work for one person may not work for another. What you place in, around, or on your body, may affect you positively or negatively.

The Federal Department of Agriculture (FDA) regulates prescribed medications, over-the-counter products, and other consumer items, including food. The FDA does <u>not</u> examine the safety of over-the-counter drugs, vitamins, and supplements like they do prescription medications. Vitamins, supplements, and over-the-counter drugs are not intended to treat, diagnose, mitigate, prevent, or cure diseases like prescribed medications.[2] Many supplements contain active ingredients that can have strong effects on the body.

The more knowledge you gain about vitamins, supplements, over-the-counter products, and prescribed medications, the easier it will be to recognize when harm comes to your body. Before my wellness journey, a physician was concerned by a slight bone density decline in my left hip and recommended that I start taking a high-level calcium supplement without asking about my calcium food intake. After taking the supplement for a week, I started having severe leg cramps at night. Thankfully, between my daily health journaling and internet research, I discovered that my leg cramps were a side effect of high calcium intake.

Once I stopped taking the calcium supplements, the leg cramps disappeared. This is one of many reasons I became 100% accountable for my health and started reading all consumer product directions, warnings, ingredients, and side effect information included with the product and on the internet. In Chapter 11, "How Your Body Communicates To You," you will gain guidance on body communication and the healing power of listening and responding.

The more you know about your body, the easier it will be to protect it from harmful recommendations and products.

YOUR 12 BODY SYSTEMS: FUNCTIONS & MAIN ORGANS[3]

As you read about your 24/7 home, plus its major parts, you'll realize your divinely-created being was beautifully designed. Once again, how you care for your 24/7 home, your daily choices, and what surrounds you, influences the health of your body, mind, and spirit. *The Human Body Atlas, by* Professor Ken Ashwell BMEDSC, MBBS, Ph.D., is a wonderful book I share in workshops to help participants become visually aware of their human body from conception to geriatric aging. You might enjoy reviewing it too. When you read about your 12 systems below, underline the functions you were not aware of. This will be a double reminder that YOU are a miracle!

YOUR NERVOUS SYSTEM is responsible for coordinating all your body functions and movements and includes your five senses: sight, touch, smell, hearing, and taste. Your three-pound brain controls your entire nervous system in unison with your spinal cord and peripheral nerves. It is the center of all your mental activity including your thoughts, learning capacity, and memory. Together with the endocrine system, your nervous system is responsible for regulating and maintaining homeostasis, your body's ability to steady and balance all physiological processes. To gain and maintain your best energy, health, and happiness, your nervous system relies on you to provide it proper hydration, clean whole foods, protection from any injury, and a balanced lifestyle.

YOUR AUTONOMIC NERVOUS SYSTEM alerts your brain and spinal cord when danger is near, informs you when changes occur within your body, regulates and controls your organs, and has the power to calm and relax you. You will not notice how it functions automatically and continuously, innervating your smooth muscle, cardiac muscle, and glands. This system can change your heart rate, breathing rate, blood pressure, body temperature, and other visceral activities that work together to maintain your body's homeostasis. It has two parts: the sympathetic nervous system, which prepares your body for stressful situations requiring energy expenditure, and the parasympathetic nervous system which slows down your heart, dilates blood vessels, decreases pupil sizes, increases digestive juices, and relaxes muscles in the gastrointestinal tract. Students who attend my therapeutic fitness classes experience their parasympathetic nervous system kicking in when they approach the final relaxation session at the end of class. The pre-relaxation session is guided with slow deep breathing, yoga, and Qigong moves, along with a grateful heart vision. Witnessing their completely relaxed state of body and mind fills my heart, especially when some of them fall asleep during this time.

YOUR CIRCULATORY SYSTEM consists of your heart, blood, and 60,000 miles of blood vessels including all your arteries, capillaries, and veins. Your heart's function is vital for your survival because it helps all the tissues in your body receive the continuous supply of the oxygen you breathe in, absorb the nutrients from your food choices, and assist in removing any metabolic waste products. A normal adult heart pumps about 5 quarts of blood every minute. When needed, your blood forms clots in response to injury, it delivers defense cells and antibodies to fight infection, contributes to your cellular metabolism, and balances (homeostasis) your fluid volume, pH, and body temperature. If you were deprived of these life necessities, your cells would undergo irreversible changes that could lead to death.

YOUR DIGESTIVE SYSTEM breaks down everything you swallow, bit by bit until the molecules are small enough to be absorbed within your body and the waste products are eliminated. The key organs include your mouth (which includes your tongue), pharynx, esophagus, stomach, intestines, pancreas, gallbladder, and liver. Your liver is your body's largest internal solid organ performing 500 different functions. Overconsumption of alcohol can damage your liver, affecting its many roles and the comfort within your body. Depending on the person and what food or drink products are consumed, it may take 24 to 72 hours or longer for consumed products to travel through the entire digestive system. What you eat, drink, and swallow is digested, absorbed, and eliminated, affecting every aspect of your brain and body. Choose wisely.

YOUR INTEGUMENTARY SYSTEM includes your nails, hair, sweat and sebaceous glands, sensory nerves, and the largest body organ, your skin. Your skin is the protective shield for your internal body to help prevent viruses, bacteria, and extreme temperatures from invading your other 11 systems. It also helps regulate your body temperature, gathers sensory information from the environment, stores water, fat, and vitamin D, and plays a role in the immune system protecting you from disease. It is about two millimeters thick and weighs approximately six pounds. Being the external body protector, your skin is the last system to receive hydration, and using lotion will help keep moisture in your skin. Where you spend most of your time is where your dead skin cells fall. A dust mite's favorite food is small pieces of dead skin flakes, hair, and dandruff that our body sheds 24 hours a day and which measures more than a teaspoon per week.[4] When I learned these interesting dust mite facts, I began changing my bedsheets and vacuuming every week.

YOUR MUSCULAR SYSTEM has more than 600 muscles, which accounts for 40 percent of your total body weight. Your muscles are attached to your bones or internal organs and blood vessels, which are responsible for voluntary physical movement. Muscles also assist with involuntary movements such as blood circulation and digestion movement. In addition to movement, muscle contraction fulfills some other important functions in the body, such as posture, joint stability, and heat production. Nearly 85 percent of the heat produced in your body is the result of muscle contraction. Your posture, such as sitting and standing, is maintained as a result of muscle contraction. Each muscle consists of skeletal muscle tissue, connective tissue, nerve tissue, and blood or vascular tissue. The more you move, the more you can groove, especially after the age of 35 when muscle loss begins in most humans. To live life to the fullest, incorporate regular and consistent joyful movement throughout your life.

YOUR SKELETAL SYSTEM consists of bones, cartilage, ligaments, and tendons which account for about 20 percent of your body weight. As a newborn, you had 270 bones and with time some of your bones unite, forming a total of 206 adult bones. Your spine is the internal sturdy frame that helps you stand upright and joins other bones to provide a protective covering for your soft organs and assists your muscles during physical movement. Your bones use oxygen, give off waste products in metabolism, and contain active tissues that consume nutrients, require a blood supply, and change shape or remodel in response to variations in mechanical stress. To help maintain stronger bones during your aging process, I encourage you to become an advocate of clean whole foods, joyful physical movement of all kinds, and weight resistance exercises. Stay strong no matter what age you become.

YOUR RESPIRATORY SYSTEM enables you to inhale oxygen to build and regenerate your body's 100 trillion cells and to exhale carbon dioxide. The main organs include your nose, nasal cavity, pharynx, larynx, trachea, and two lungs. Your lungs, some of the largest organs in your body, along with the help of your diaphragm muscle, can breathe in 21,000 times a day, enough to oxygenate the 1800+ gallons of blood pumped throughout your circulatory system each day. Breathing in quality air and regular physical movement is important for maintaining a healthy respiratory system.

YOUR ENDOCRINE SYSTEM houses hormones, the chemical substances that control activities in all your body tissues, which are released by this system and controlled by your pituitary gland. Growth, development, metabolism, and homeostasis are its primary functions. The endocrine system's main organs include the thyroid, adrenals, pancreas, pineal body, ovaries, or testes. Stress and poor food choices can negatively affect this system as well as all your other 11 systems as you will read in Chapter 7, "Stress Can Do What To Me??!!"

YOUR REPRODUCTIVE SYSTEM and those of your children were divinely designed to be honored, loved, and protected. According to the Centers for Disease Control and Prevention (CDC), "Congenital syphilis, an incredibly harmful infection and sexually transmitted disease (STD) has increased a staggering 279% since 2015," while other harmful STDs increased from 20% - 70%.[5] With males and females having different organs producing reproductive cells, all of them require a grounded relationship to honor themselves and each other throughout life. Females provide the human environment for an embryo to develop, along with the body's ovaries, fallopian tubes, uterus, and vagina. When a female becomes pregnant, she is the one who walks the road of nurturing her unborn child and deserves a supportive and loving spouse to walk this parental journey with her. Male reproductive organs include testes, ductus deferens, seminal vesicle, prostate gland, and penis.

Today, the U.S. STD rates continue to climb rapidly. This proves that many people are on a road to self-harm and will suffer consequences, including those involved in their lives. All of this is due to selfish pleasure seeking. Not until a person opens their mind and heart to honor, respect, and truly love themselves and others will this downward spiral reverse. Parents and all adults, I hope you will claim your role to teach our children to honor, love, and respect themselves throughout their lives.

YOUR URINARY SYSTEM is important because it maintains the balance of water and electrolytes in your blood and excretes liquid waste and toxins from your body. Its main organs include your two kidneys, urethra, and bladder. The kidneys filter waste materials from all the food, drinks, over-the-counter drugs, medications, and toxic substances brought into your body. The kidneys also make hormones that help control your blood pressure, create red blood cells, and assist in the health and strength of your bones.

As you continue to read throughout this book, you will learn how important it is to become knowledgeable of all foods and drinks you consume. In Chapter 8, "Your Food Choices Matter," you will gain tips about how food can positively and negatively affect your body. I hope that this book will be a guide if you experience negative symptoms in your urinary system or any other body system. Once again, reading the side effects of all prescriptions, over-the-counter drugs, supplements, and vitamins is helpful because your kidneys process these products and can be affected by all of them.

YOUR IMMUNE / LYMPHATIC SYSTEM protects and fights off diseases within your body. All immune cells come from precursors in the bone marrow and develop into mature cells through a series of changes that can occur in different parts of your body. The many parts consist of your skin, bone marrow, bloodstream, lymph vessels, 500-600 lymph nodes, thymus, spleen, and mucosal tissue. Simple and regular hand washing is important in protecting you from germs, viruses, and bacteria. Having a balanced life helps to strengthen your immune system.[6]

As you will learn in this book, a wellness journey helps you grow in self-knowledge and self-respect and to be true to what you want in life. You will learn how your daily choices affect you either positively or negatively. Becoming aware of how you feel is vital to regulating your wellness. If stress creeps into your life, pay close attention to all the aspects revealed on your **Life Balance Foundation** scores. This may help you discover which areas are causing discomfort or stress in your body, mind, and spirit. Once you are aware of the causes, you can decide what to remove, or include, so you can reach your goals.

Another aspect that causes a change in your body, mind, and spirit is the aging process. The National Institute of Aging has conducted ongoing research to identify the interactions among genetic, environmental, lifestyle, behavioral, and social factors and their influence on the initiation and progression of age-related diseases and degenerative conditions.

To learn more about the aging process go to their website: **https://www.nia.nih.gov/**.

CHAPTER 7

Stress Can Do *What* to Me!!??

The time to relax is when you think you have no time.

Stress contributes up to 80% of all primary care physician visits in the United States and is known to cause poor choices that sabotage one's best intentions.[1]

This cat resembles how I felt before and during my health decline. Before waking up to the light, all my daily choices and thought processes contributed to my health decline. I was very weak when it came to living an intentional lifestyle but very strong in working seven days a week in the medical

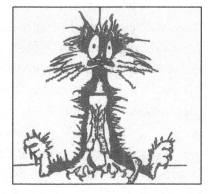

profession and eating on the run. Stress had a constant green light in my life due to low levels of self-respect, self-love, and protective boundaries. It affected the quality of my sleep, time management, health, life, and spiritual balance.

On top of all this, the three unexpected life challenges appeared in my life from nowhere! For eight months I felt like a mummy walking in a daze. Not until an adventure hiking trip to Sedona, Arizona, and the Grand Canyon did I feel an ounce of relief. On the first day of hiking, I could feel nature's healing powers as I breathed in the fresh western air. Rays of sunshine beamed on my body, and the sacred soil touched my feet as I walked with my dear friends, Paula and Suzanne. Connecting with God's nature and being with loving friends helped lift the eight months of heavy stress and lingering grief that was stuck in my soul.

What led me to this healing adventure was a simple glance at my church bulletin two weeks after my dad's death. There in small print, I read about Reverend Carl Malm, Executive Director of Huntsville Association of Pastoral (HAPC) and the Center of Loss, Grief, and Change was offering a series of three classes on dealing with grief at a local church. Without hesitation, I attended the first class along with a couple of hospice chaplains and five people who had lost loved ones. As they shared their feelings of loss and sadness, I began to understand that I was experiencing normal responses to grief, something I had never felt before. Attending those classes was a true gift from God because they offered me lessons and wisdom I needed at that time. To continue the lessons of grief, I now celebrate my father on his birthday with a nature hike or a celebration with my family.

If you ever experience loss and grief in any form, do yourself a favor and reach out for help, guidance, and comfort. Dr. Elisabeth Kubler-Ross, the author of *Death and Dying* and many other books, has been a leader in grief and healing. Learning how to grieve is an essential step to healing and releasing stress so you can reclaim your energy, health, and happiness.

Personality type and pride levels can also create stress havoc within a person's body, mind, and spirit. Why was I so compelled to work seven days a week, especially after my entire world had turned upside down from all these losses in life? I later discovered my "Type A" personality helped me become a master at covering up the large hole of emptiness in my unbalanced life as I walked around in a cloak of professional pride. Taking a deep look in the mirror helped me understand the tight hold I had on worldly things, outward success, and internal fear. Seeing my reflection revealed my personal desire to control my life instead of allowing God's plan for my life.

When your stress levels rise, what do you reach for? Is it the typical things most people choose? Chocolate, a sweet treat, or a soda? Did you know "stressed" spelled backward is DESSERTS? Or do you need salty foods like chips or fast food, alcohol, medications, cigarettes, vaping, or illegal drugs to help you relax and unwind? Unfortunately, reaching for these items does just the opposite for your body, mind, and spirit. They begin to ignite endless cravings that can lead to addiction.

Like Satan's deceitfulness with Eve, the food, alcohol, medication, and illegal drug industries encourage you to pick their products from their trees. As it was for Eve in the garden, we humans struggle with obedience when temptation lures us. It all begins with the least amount of thought or awareness. What's one little taste going to hurt? Are we just trying to calm ourselves down from stress, or is it the enticing pleasure that keeps us running to all those unhealthy choices?

As stated in an article, "Sugar and Dopamine: The Link Between Sweets and Addiction," published by the Wellness

Retreat and Recovery Center in San Jose, California, "Alcohol has a high sugar content, so alcoholics' bodies and brains are adjusted to a high level of sugar from daily or frequent drinking. When alcoholics get sober, the brain loses out of the daily sugar rush it is accustomed to from drinking. This can create intense sugar cravings, and many alcoholics report overconsumption of candy and sweets during this adjustment period." The same can be said for recovering drug addicts.

An animal study in the medical journal, *PLOS One*, titled "Intense Sweetness Surpasses Cocaine Reward" reported that the pleasure of sweet taste outweighs the pleasure from cocaine.[2] Wow!!! If we humans are anything like these animals, it goes to prove why humans reach for pleasure foods and other brain-altering products for stress relief. No wonder our nation has seen a rise in obesity in adults and children since the early 1970s.[3] The rise in obesity contributes to many preventable diseases including heart disease, diabetes, and cancer.[4]

Let's take a deeper look at four stress factors that contribute to energy depletion, human pain, and disease.

FOUR MAJOR STRESS FACTORS

CHEMICAL STRESS

Environmental chemicals such as air pollution, smoke, pesticides, herbicides, air fresheners, and cleaning products used in and around your home and work environment can create stress in your body. Pumping gas in a car also exposes one to toxic gas fumes. Chemical stress is present in food and drink products containing controversial ingredients, such as pesticides used in farming and the added hormones and antibiotics used in meat factory farming processes.[5] In Chapter 10, "Clean Is Supreme," you will learn about controversial ingredients, other chemicals used in our food industry, and how they affect your body.

EMOTIONAL STRESS

Life situations that may cause you feelings of anger, sadness, fear, regret, anxiety, guilt, low self-esteem, and grief can contribute to your stress levels. Losing something of value, gaining more than you can handle, feeling disrespected, or a loss of control can be difficult challenges and make recovery difficult.

MENTAL STRESS

Mental stress may be caused by any life situation that demands more than you can handle at the time. For example, when the 2019 COVID pandemic first appeared and reignited two years later, it created political, personal, relationship, business, church, school, and financial difficulties beyond anyone's control. Many have been affected by sickness and the loss of loved ones.[6]

PHYSICAL STRESS

Nature, public services, and work environments can contribute to stress when weather fluctuations, temperature changes, ventilation, noise, vibration, and low energy radiation occur. This can cause physical changes within your muscular, skeletal, cardiovascular, and nervous systems, and affect your body's hematologic, immune, and cell chemistry values.[7,8,9]

TIPS TO RELIEVE STRESS

Think about which factor(s) are creating stress in your life at the moment. Write them down in a journal and release your feelings on paper as if you were talking with your best friend.

When stress develops from any factor, our body goes through changes alerting our adrenal glands to produce cortisol, known as the "stress hormone." Occasional stress is not that bad on our body. In fact, sometimes it's good for us. However, if you have chronic stress, your entire body is constantly flooded with cortisol causing negative symptoms and cravings that lead to overeating processed foods, consuming alcohol or drugs, and indulging in mindless habits. All of this depletes your energy, health, and happiness. Reflect on these questions regarding stressful days:

- What do I typically eat and drink?
- How are my moods and sleep?
- How much internet, social media, and TV do I absorb during these times?
- How many daily hours and weekdays do I work?
- What do I typically do to ease my stress level?

Replacing negative habits with positive ones will lead you to the Metanoia path. As you begin walking a wellness journey, release your thoughts from your heart and mind every day. Lace up your tennis shoes and enjoy some joyful physical movement in the fresh air and nature. Find a quiet space and begin mindful breathing. Play peaceful music wherever you are. State three things you are most grateful for each day. These simple actions will help you calm down, relax, and release stress to prevent destruction from entering your body, mind, and spirit.

CHAPTER 8

Your Food Choices Matter

*The food you choose can be your best medicine
or your slowest poison.*

Your daily food choices are how your body receives fuel for growth, development, energy, immunity, and every body function. The more knowledge you gain about food, the wiser choices you can make for yourself and your family.

An interesting fact most people don't think about is how they were introduced to food and why they like or dislike certain kinds. Your official introduction started when your father's sperm joined with your mother's embryo. Your parents' choices of food, drinks, and other substances they consumed before and at the time of your conception created a foundation within you. Their nutritional habits and overall health influenced your development. What your mother ate, drank, and consumed while she was pregnant went into fueling your body, mind, and spirit. In addition to your parents, other adults, the schools you attended, and even your friends may have influenced your food choices.

Take a moment and think about the food and drinks you enjoyed when you were a child and what you enjoy today. Can you see a correlation? Do you crave any childhood foods or have emotional connections to them? If so, your answers are offering you self-awareness.

Your food and drink choices, combined with your **Life Balance Foundation** scores, are major factors in the quality of your present wellness.

Along with balancing your life, this food plate is a simple prescription for your wellness journey. The more you open your mind and heart to understanding how food affects your total being, the easier you can make the best choices. Consuming a daily variety of whole colorful food, along with water and healthy fats, provides your body, mind, and spirit the best fuel.

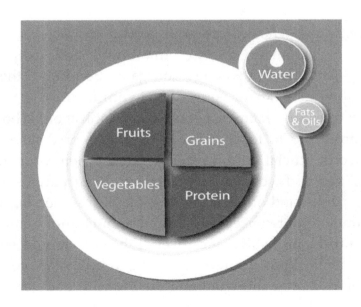

KNOW YOUR MACRONUTRIENTS

The main food categories are called **Macronutrients,** better known as **Carbohydrates, Proteins**, and **Fats.** All foods in these categories have energizing chemical substances that sustain and maintain your life. Let's take a deeper look at what foods are in each of these categories and what they do for you.

CARBOHYDRATES

Carbohydrates are primarily found in whole fruits, vegetables, and grains that consist of plant fiber, starch, and sugar (fructose, sucrose, glucose). Another carbohydrate source, dairy products, contains milk sugar (lactose).

In this chapter, I will focus on colorful whole plant foods, a highly nutritious food source, yet the lowest consumed foods in the United States. It amazed me to learn potatoes and tomatoes are the highest consumed vegetables in the United States. Why do you think this is? They are used to prepare two of the highest consumed fast foods in the U.S, French fries and pizza sauce.[1]

At the beginning of my wellness journey, it made sense to me to consume more whole colorful vegetables because they are low in calories, contain healing properties, and provide the best energy boost.

The U.S. Forestry Service revealed amazing information about the power of consuming plants in their *Medical Botany* article:[2] "Our earliest human ancestors found plants to heal wounds, cure diseases, and ease troubled minds. People on all continents have long used hundreds, if not thousands, of indigenous plants, for treatment of various ailments dating back to prehistory. Knowledge about the healing properties or poisonous effects of plants, mineral salts, and herbs accumulated from these earliest times to provide health and predates all other medical treatment."

Susan J. Zunino, an Agricultural Research Service molecular biologist, led nutrition-focused research that resulted in these first-ever findings: "Rosemary, the fragrant herb that enlivens roast chicken and other favorites, and turmeric, the mainstay spice of curry dishes, contain powerful natural compounds that, in test tubes, can kill cells of childhood cancer. What's more, grapes, strawberries, and other familiar fruits—and some vegetables—also have chemicals that can destroy the cells of this cancer, known as "acute lymphoblastic leukemia."[3]

It was also interesting to learn: "A full 40 percent of the drugs behind the pharmacist's counter in the Western world are derived from plants that people have used for centuries, including the top 20 best-selling prescription drugs in the United States today."[4] This proves food can be your best medicine, and the choice is all yours.

Some of the health-boosting benefits your body receives from phytochemicals, the natural chemicals of plants include:

- ANTIOXIDANTS help remove potentially dangerous oxidizing agents from your body.
- ANTI-INFLAMMATORY properties reduce inflammation in the body that shows up in many diseases.
- ANTI-BACTERIAL properties combat bacteria in the body.
- ANTI-FUNGAL properties help prevent fungal growth that weakens the immune system.

Plants with more fiber and starch are classified as **complex carbohydrates**, and plants such as fruit with more natural sugar (sucrose, glucose, and fructose) are classified as **simple carbohydrates**.

Complex carbohydrates benefit your digestion process and their starch helps suppress your appetite. The plant's fiber can increase your frequency of bowel movements, lower glucose and cholesterol levels, reduce calorie intake, and help prevent cardiovascular disease. Whole plant foods with high fiber include beans, fruits, nuts, peas, vegetables, seeds, and whole grains.[5]

Your body loves whole vegetables, fruits, and grains because they offer your body quick energy from their natural sugar base compared to protein and fat food sources. If anyone tells you to stop eating so many carbs, they are mainly referring to processed foods filled with added sugar and controversial ingredients, not whole vegetables, fruits, or whole grains.

A simple example of whole food vs. processed food is an orange and a glass of orange juice. Eating an orange offers your body more stabilizing nutrition compared to drinking a cup of orange juice. Orange juice has more calories, more sugar content, and less nutritious fiber.

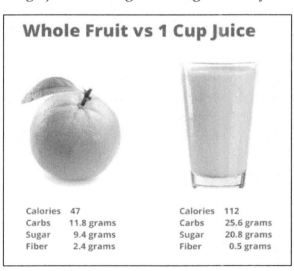

Whole Fruit vs 1 Cup Juice

Calories	47		Calories	112
Carbs	11.8 grams		Carbs	25.6 grams
Sugar	9.4 grams		Sugar	20.8 grams
Fiber	2.4 grams		Fiber	0.5 grams

Complex carbohydrates, especially whole grains, offer more health benefits than the popular processed grain foods such as crackers, chips, pasta, bread, cereals, and snack bars responsible for many glucose highs and crashes in your body.

Like I used to be before my wellness journey, most people do not know the nutritional value of eating whole grains. Whole grains contain all three parts of the seed, also known as the kernel. The seed has three parts: the endosperm, bran, and germ. Whole grains are healthier, provide more protein, fiber, and important vitamins and minerals. When grain is processed to make foods like cereals, pasta, bread, and flour, the refining process normally removes the bran and germ, leaving only the endosperm. Without the bran and germ, about 25% of the grain's protein is lost, and the content of other nutrients is significantly reduced.[6] If you would like to learn more about whole grains, their health benefits, and see some nutritious recipes, go to the Whole Grain Council website: www.wholegrainscouncil.org. This is an excellent resource!

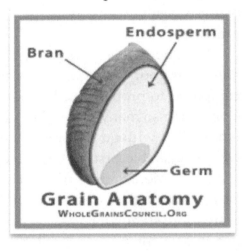

Grain Anatomy
WholeGrainsCouncil.Org

PROTEIN

Protein, another important macronutrient, is found in plants, fish, and animals. When whole protein food sources are consumed, their nutrients help support many body functions, including:

- Protein is necessary for every cell in your body to help sustain proper growth and development, especially in childhood, adolescence, and pregnancy.
- Protein helps your body build and repair cells and body tissue: epithelial, connective, muscle, and nervous.
- Protein is also a major source of energy. However, when you consume too much protein it becomes stored energy for later needs unless your body is already filled with energy consumed from carbohydrates. If this is the case, any extra protein not used for stored energy will turn into fat.
- Protein is a major part of your skin, hair, nails, muscle, bone, and internal organs. It is also found in almost all your body fluids.
- Protein is essential for many body processes, such as vision, immune response, fluid balance, blood clotting, production of hormones, antibodies, and enzymes.[7]

Protein provides many more functions for your body, although knowing the major sources I share on the next page may inspire you to make healthier protein choices.

HOW MUCH PROTEIN SHOULD I CONSUME EACH DAY?

There is ongoing research about the amount of daily protein you need, and it depends on your specific body facts including your age, weight, and activity level. Today, the U.S. Food and Drug

Administration (FDA) recommends an "average" of 50 grams of protein per day from a variety of protein foods. To learn your specific recommended daily macronutrient needs, visit the United States Department of Agriculture (USDA) and check out the Daily Reference Intake Calculator (DRI Calculator) @ **https://www.nal.usda.gov/fnic/dri-calculator/**.[8]

This data represents the most current scientific knowledge on specific nutrient needs. However, individual requirements may be higher or lower than the DRI recommendations.

After reviewing the USDA DRI Calculator for micronutrient food gram recommendations, take a look at the quick protein list below that I created at the beginning of my wellness journey.[9] This list made it easier for me to choose a variety of daily protein sources.

PROTEIN SAMPLE AND GRAM LIST

1 cup tuna	54 grams
1 cup chicken breast	43 grams
1 cup salmon	40 grams
1 cup Greek yogurt	25 grams
1 cup black beans	15 grams
¼ cup pumpkin seeds	9 grams
1 cup green peas	8 grams
1 egg	6 grams
1 cup spinach	5 grams
2 TBSP almonds	2.5 grams
1 cup broccoli	2 grams

Were you surprised to see the plant-based foods and Greek yogurt on this protein food sample list?

I've also included a *Micronutrient for Wellness* list at the end of this chapter to help you learn about specific vitamins and minerals in foods and how they enhance your health.

FAT

Fat is found in both plant and animal sources. It has nine calories per gram, five more calories than a gram of protein or carbohydrate foods, so you need to be careful about your daily fat consumption to maintain a healthy weight. Fats have many important body roles including:[10]

- Fat stores energy above what the body needs and serves as a secondary energy source once calories from carbohydrates are used up.
- Fat is a basic foundation of your cell membranes and is necessary for growth and development.
- Fat supports key body processes in your nervous system, reproduction, immune response, and blood clotting.
- Fat helps the body absorb important fat-soluble vitamins (A, D, E, and K) and plays a major role in your cholesterol levels.
- Fat is vital to maintain the health of your skin and hair.
- Fat in food provides taste and consistency and helps you feel full.

Fat constitutes the bulk of your dry brain mass so it's wise to choose nutritious, healthy fat foods because your body does not produce essential fats by itself.[11]

The American Heart Association (AHA) recommends consuming foods rich in monosaturated and polyunsaturated fats and to limit or avoid saturated or trans fats that lead to heart disease and stroke.[12] To learn more about healthy fats, check out the American Heart Association website @ **www.heart.org** and Dr. Daniel Amen's website @ **www.amensclinic.com**. Dr. Amen was one of my favorite instructors at the Institute of Integrative

Nutrition and is a leader in brain health. He too promotes healthy nutrition and life balance for the best life.

Below is a quick guide to help you incorporate healthier fats into your meals and see which foods to limit or avoid for the best energy, health, and happiness.

FOODS WITH HEALTHY FAT

Contain healthy monosaturated and polyunsaturated fats

- Oils (Canola, Olive, Peanut, Sesame, and Safflower)
- Fatty fish (Salmon, Mackerel, Tuna, Herring, Sardines, Trout)
- Nuts and Seeds (Flaxseed, Walnuts, Sunflower seeds)
- Avocados

UNHEALTHY FAT FOODS

Contain unhealthy saturated fats and hydrogenated oils

- Beef, Pork, and Chicken fat (limit)
- Butter and Cheese (limit)
- Coconut oil, Palm Kernel, and Palm oils (avoid)
- Fried foods (avoid)
- Margarine and partially hydrogenated oils (avoid)
- Pastries, Crackers, Cookies, and Snack food (avoid)

How are your healthy fat food choices compared to the unhealthy fat foods to limit or avoid?

To help bring in the good food choices and to release the bad, incorporating at least one new nutritious food per week will introduce you to new tastes and body sensations. Before long, you will recognize new favorites, learn to tolerate others due to their nutrition benefits, and some you may not like at all. Awareness of the health benefits of all the whole foods you consume will help you obtain your goals.

Another favorite instructor, while I attended the Institute of Integrative Nutrition, is Dr. Joel Furhman. Dr. Furhman has guided many people to disease reversal, including me. He taught me the importance of food's nutritional value in his lectures and two of his books, *Eat To Live* and *The End of Diabetes.*

On the next page, is a **High Nutritious Foods** list I created at the beginning of my wellness journey and recently adapted to point out high oxalate foods you will read about in this chapter's section, "Overdoing A Good Thing." This list made it easier for me to fill in my meal plate sections as I incorporated a variety of new nutritious foods. There are many more fruit and vegetable choices you can add to this list. Please be aware, if you overeat high oxalate foods you may experience body discomforts and some serious health problems including kidney stones.

HIGH NUTRITIOUS FOODS

Fruits	Vegetables	Whole Grains	Proteins	Fats
Blueberries	Kale, Spinach *	Quinoa	Chicken Breast	Avocado *
Strawberries	Mustard, Collard Greens*	Oats	Salmon/Sardines/Halibut/Tuna	Sesame Oil
Blackberries	Watercress, Arugula	Rye	Beans/Lentils *	Virgin Olive Oil
Raspberries	Swiss Chard	Corn, Popcorn	Greek Yogurt	Salmon, Trout
Cranberries	Bok Choy	Brown Rice (colored)*	Egg Whites	Sardines, Mackerel
Grapes	Blackeye Peas	Amaranth	Cottage Cheese	Albacore tuna
Cantaloupe	Romaine Lettuce	Barley *	Many Vegetables	Nuts *
Orange *	Brussel Sprouts, Cabbage	Buckwheat *	Seeds: pumpkin, sesame, sunflower	Flax seeds
Peaches	Garlic, Mushrooms, Onion	Sorghum	Nuts: almonds, pecan, walnut *	Sunflower Seeds
Apple	Broccoli	Teff	Beef, Turkey, Pork	Pumpkin seeds
Mango	Green Peas, Carrots *	Triticale	Whole Grains	Soybeans *
High Oxalates *	High Oxalates *	High Oxalates *	High Oxalates *	High Oxalates *

MICRONUTRIENTS FOR WELLNESS

Micronutrients are the actual minerals and vitamins from the carbohydrates, proteins, and fats you chose to consume. Vitamins are naturally present in plant and animal food products. Minerals are substances found naturally in the soil and water absorbed by plants, which are then eaten by humans and animals. Keep in mind that the quality of the soil and water absorbed by plants is transported into the humans and animals who eat them. Just like the food you eat and your life balance, the source of the plant's nutrients and environment determines their health. You will learn more about this in Chapter 10, "Clean Is Supreme."

According to the FDA, many people in the U.S. have low levels of iron, potassium, calcium, and vitamin D which leads to high blood pressure, osteoporosis, and anemia.[13] Eating a variety of whole nutritious foods rich in varied vitamins and minerals provides a person with healthier growth, development, and improved body function.

At the beginning of my wellness journey, I researched the vitamins and minerals in food and how they could empower my health. This knowledge helped me implement more varied colorful plant foods, healthier proteins, and fats into my day. The research also revealed that my body was lacking in Magnesium, so I purchased pepita seeds and other magnesium enriched foods at the grocery store to see what would happen after I consumed them. With a heart filled with hope and more home cooking, within a short time, I was able to eliminate my blood pressure and thyroid medications. This proved to me that food can be the best medicine when combined with a balanced life.

In the next few pages, you will see the **Micronutrients For Wellness** lists that consist of 27 major micronutrients, the body functions they help provide, and some top food sources for each. When you compare your present health status to each micronutrient body function on this list, you may discover a variety of foods you can implement to improve your energy, health, and happiness.

If you presently have issues with any of the body functions listed, review the food nutrients for that micronutrient. Are you consuming any of these whole foods regularly? If not, now is a good time to try them. If you'd like to see additional foods for each micronutrient, try an internet web search for foods per micronutrient. It's amazing how YOU CAN empower your body, mind, and spirit with nutritious food choices.

MICRONUTRIENTS FOR WELLNESS

MICRONUTRIENT	WHAT IT DOES	SOME TOP FOOD SOURCES
Vitamin A	Vision Red blood cell formation Immune function Skin and bone formation Reproduction Growth and development	Sweet Potato, Spinach, Carrots, Herring, Broccoli, Green leafy vegetables, Red Peppers Cantaloupe, Mango, Pumpkin, Cheese, Milk, Eggs
B1 Thiamin	Converts food into energy Nervous system function	Black beans, Mussels, Acorn squash, Sunflower seeds, Peas, Corn, Nuts, Whole grains, Trout, Tuna, Yogurt
B2 Riboflavin	Converts food into energy Growth and development Red blood cell formation	Mushrooms, Almonds, Blueberries, Kidney beans, Sunflower seeds, Pork, Cheese, Milk
B3 Niacin	Digestion Converts food into energy Cholesterol production Nervous system function	Beans, Legumes, Peanuts, Whole grains, Seafood, Poultry, Pork, Beef, Eggs, Milk
B5 Pantothenic Acid	Fat metabolism Hormone production Generates energy from food Nervous system function Red blood cell production	Avocados, Sunflower seeds, Beans, Mushrooms, Peas, Sweet Potato, Legumes, Corn, Peanuts, Hazelnuts, Whole grains, Yogurt, Cheese, Trout, Chicken, Pork, Turkey, Beef, Eggs, Milk
B6	Immune Function Red blood cell function Nervous system function Macronutrient metabolism	Beans, Garlic, Chickpeas, Peanuts, Russet potatoes, Fruits (other than citrus), Salmon, Tuna, Turkey, Beef, Pork
B7 Biotin	Energy storage Macronutrient metabolism	Avocados, Fruits, Raspberries, Cauliflower, Whole grains, Liver, Pork, Salmon
B9 Folate	Red blood cell reproduction Protein metabolism Prevention of birth defects	Pink and black beans, Soybeans, Black-eyed peas, Edamame, Asparagus, Peanuts, Beets, Okra, Spinach, Hazelnuts, Boysenberries, Almonds, Oranges, Broccoli
B12	Red Blood cell formation Nervous system function Convert foods to energy	Oysters, Mussels, Crab, Herring, Trout, Salmon, Pork, Beef, Lamb, Cheese

Choline	Brain development Metabolism Cell signaling Fat transport and metabolism Liver function Muscle movement Nerve function	Black beans, Cauliflower, Spinach, Black-eyed peas, Peas, Carrots, Lima beans, Soybeans, Corn, Broccoli, Tomatoes, Eggs, Pork, Beef, Oyster, Flounder Turkey, Chicken
Vitamin C	Wound healing Immune function Collagen formation Connective tissue formation Antioxidant	Peppers, Strawberries, Blueberries, Currants, Citrus fruits, Kiwi, Cantaloupe, Brussel sprouts, Cauliflower, Collards, Garlic, Turnip greens, Kale, Spinach, Broccoli, Cabbage, Peas, Asparagus, Spinach, Tomatoes, Soybeans, Lima Beans, Mango
Vitamin D	Blood pressure regulation Immune function Hormone Production Calcium balance Bone growth Nervous system function	Mushrooms, Mackerel, Trout, Flounder, Salmon, Herring, Sardines, Tuna, Fish oil, Cod liver oil, Pork, Eggs
Vitamin E	Immune function Antioxidant Blood vessel formation	Sunflower seeds, Almonds, Hazelnuts, Peanuts, Turnip greens, Spinach, Asparagus, Winter squash, Kiwi, Sweet potato, Broccoli, Peanut butter, Vegetable oils
Vitamin K	Blood clotting Strong bones	Kale, Spinach, Broccoli, Peas, Mustard greens, Celery, Collards, Turnip greens, Green beans, Beet greens, Swiss chard, Cabbage, Kiwi, Blueberries, Soybeans, Endive
Calcium	Bone and teeth formation Hormone secretion Muscle contraction Nervous system function Blood vessel constriction and relaxation Blood clotting	Almonds, Kale, Collard greens, Soybeans, Turnip greens, Black beans, Salmon, Sardines, Yogurt, Cheese, Milk
Chloride	Digestion Fluid balance Nervous system function Food to energy conversion Acid-base balance	Celery, Lettuce, Tomatoes, Olives, Seaweed, Rye, Sea Salt, Table salt
Chromium	Insulin function Macronutrient metabolism	Broccoli, Basil, Garlic, Green beans, Oranges, Apples, Bananas, Grapes, Whole grains, Turkey

Copper	Antioxidant Energy production Iron metabolism Bone formation Nervous system function Collagen formation Connective tissue formation	Beans, Lentils, Nuts, Cocoa powder, Potatoes, Dark leafy green vegetables, Prunes, Black pepper, Yeast, Whole grains Oysters, Shellfish, Liver
Iodine	Metabolism Thyroid hormone function Reproduction function Growth and development	Seaweed, Seafood, Ionized salt, Potatoes, Whole grains, Dairy products, Turkey
Iron	Energy production Immune function Wound healing Reproduction Red blood cell formation Growth and development	Sunflower seeds, Pumpkin seeds, Kale, Soybeans, Collard greens, Broccoli, Spinach, Peas, Green vegetables, Nuts, Beans, Blueberries, Prunes, Raisins, Whole grains, Seafood, Poultry, Eggs
Magnesium	Energy production Immune function Muscle contraction Nerve system function Blood pressure regulation Hormone secretion Bones and teeth formation Blood sugar regulation Normal heart rhythm Protein formation	Pumpkin seeds, Sunflower seeds, Almonds, Peanuts, Hazelnuts, Black beans, Soybeans, Spinach, Lima beans, Black-eyed peas, Squash, Bananas, Raisins, Russet potatoes, Whole grains
Manganese	Wound healing Cartilage and bone formation Macronutrient metabolism	Pumpkin seeds, Sunflower seeds, Blueberries, Almonds, Black Beans, Soybeans, Beets, Black-eyed peas, Lima beans, Pineapple, Spinach, Sweet potato, Whole grains
Molybdenum	Enzyme production	Beans, Peas, Nuts, Whole grains
Phosphorous	Bone formation Energy production and storage Hormone activation Acid-base balance	Beans, Peas, Almonds, Peanuts, Sunflower seeds, Pumpkin seeds, Whole grains, Cheese, Poultry, Salmon, Cod, Pork

Selenium	Immune function Thyroid function Reproduction Antioxidant	Sunflower seeds, Nuts, Whole grains, Salmon, Herring, Oysters, Flounder, Tuna, Turkey, Cheese
Sodium	Blood pressure regulation Nervous system function Acid-base balance Muscle contraction Fluid balance	Beets, Celery, Cheese, Chicken, Milk, Processed foods, Sodium products
Zinc	Immune function Nervous system function Wound healing Protein formation Reproduction Taste and smell Growth and development	Black beans, Sunflower seeds, Pumpkin seeds, Almonds, Whole grains, Beef, Lamb, Oysters, Turkey

You gain a new set of talents and skills when you open your mind and taste buds to new nutritious foods. It's interesting how different foods taste depending on the way they are prepared or cooked. Raw fruits and vegetables are an easy fix. Sautéing, steaming, baking, or roasting in an oven are simple ways to cook them.

In addition to the recipes in Chapter 17, "Simple Nutritious Recipes," the internet is a great resource for new ways to prepare food. You will discover new favorites when you try a variety of whole plant foods and new protein sources rather than relying on those regular processed and fast-food choices.

If cooking is not your thing, you can obtain whole-cooked foods from grocery stores that offer nutritious food bars or restaurants that focus on offering clean whole foods. The most nutritious energy snacks come in the form of fresh whole fruits, vegetables, whole grains, nuts, and seeds. Have fun and try them all! Transforming your life is a step-by-step and day-by-day process. It helps to practice, practice, practice to accomplish your goals! If you stumble and get off the wellness path, pick yourself up, dust yourself off, forgive yourself, reset, refuel your spirit, and get back on the Metanoia path with consistent discipline and perseverance. I've had to do this many times.

Just like the sticky note goal reminders, keep this food plate and the *Macronutrient List* in your memory, on your refrigerator, and near your pantry. YOU CAN make it happen!

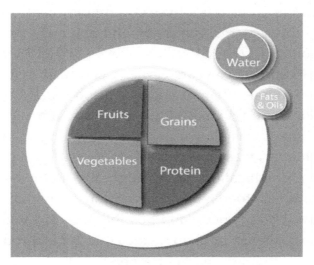

OVERDOING A GOOD THING

As she gently smiled, my physician kindly said, "Your labs look good but your iron and LDLs are a little on the high side." Without any thought, I shouted "What!" How in the world can a healthy and physically active Integrative Nutrition Health Coach have this revealed on her lab reports? My physician did not explain why the lab numbers had increased from last year's physical. She had no idea. It was totally up to me to figure out why.

During the previous year, I had purposely increased my daily volume of Vitamin C and carotene foods (mainly red peppers, citrus fruits, sweet potatoes, and carrots) to enhance my immune system and body functions. And, to increase my muscle mass, I doubled my boiled egg consumption. I thought that if I consumed more powerhouse foods, my health benefits would increase. Boy, was I WRONG!

Once home from this physician appointment, my priority was to sit down at the computer and research the causes of elevated iron and LDL (cholesterol) levels. What I learned took me by surprise because years earlier I had read that Vitamin C was a water-soluble vitamin and when too much is consumed, the extra Vitamin C will naturally excrete through our urine. This made me think it was okay if I accidentally consumed too much Vitamin C foods. I was misled and WRONG! All the professional experience and education never taught me that consuming too much Vitamin C foods could create an excess of high iron absorption within my body and possibly lead to a toxic disorder called hemochromatosis. I had no idea that hemochromatosis can cause damage to many parts of a person's body, including the liver, heart, pancreas, endocrine glands, and joints, if it is not prevented or treated.[14,15,16] This new education was a mind opener and a big lesson in overdoing a good thing.

As I continued my research, I was shocked to learn just one large egg offered 275 mg of cholesterol, more than a day's worth of cholesterol. Oh, my goodness! And there I was eating at least two eggs a day for the protein that comes from the white of the egg, not the yolk. One study[17] recommended limiting dietary cholesterol to less than 200 mg because dietary cholesterol, including egg yolks, is harmful to our arteries, the blood vessels that deliver oxygen-rich blood from the heart to the tissues of the body. My goodness, there was so much I needed to learn when it came to recommended portion sizes, even with the most nutritious foods.

Thankfully, the following year's physical lab report revealed that my cholesterol was within the normal range. Although, this past year's yearly physical lab reports revealed three irregularities going on in my body: Low iron, blood in my urine, and arrhythmia. Once again, my physician was very kind and started with the positives and then told me the three negatives. "What!" I shouted again, and with more bewilderment than ever. "How could this be?" I asked. She asked me if I felt weak or dizzy. "No, not at all," I responded. She told me I needed to see a urologist and cardiologist to determine if there had been any damage to my urinary system or heart.

Six weeks later, I met with her again to review the urologist's report and to share my research results. Unfortunately, she could not pull up the report on the computer, so I shared his comments with her. She heard me repeat the urologist's comments as he walked into my patient waiting room, "Hi! I have great news! You do not have bladder cancer." I told him that bladder cancer was not a concern of mine as I had researched what I think created blood in my urine. I handed him the printed resources which explained consuming plant foods with high levels of oxalates can result in blood in urine, anemia, and arrhythmia in addition to many more diseases.

Oxalates are compounds found in a large range of plant foods and when consumed at a high level for a person's unique body chemistry, can become an antinutrient.[18] I told him what I ate on most days and foods I had added four months prior. The high oxalate foods I usually ate included almonds, pecans, walnuts, chard, collards, beets, beet greens, soybeans, sweet potatoes, and bananas. The foods I had added four months earlier were English cucumbers, which can cause harm to the urinary system, and figs, which can cause anemia.

Without looking at the reports, he handed them back to me, and said, "I don't believe food can do that to you." I said, "In 2014, I reversed the disease in my body by changing my nutrition, and I'm writing a book about it." He asked, "Did you lose any weight when you reversed the disease?" "Yes," I responded and added, "About 10 pounds." Looking straight into my eyes he said: "That's what did it. I don't believe food has anything to do with reversing disease." Whoa, this very popular urologist just stepped on my passion strings, and I responded, "I believe it does!"

As I handed my physician the same research information I tried to share with the urologist, she said I needed to get all the cardiovascular tests recommendations completed. "If all your tests come back normal, we will say you are healthy and put you on some medicine." she said.

I responded, "It will take some time to turn this around, and I do not take medicine." She peered at me as if I was a disobedient child, although what she heard and saw was my determination to find out what was going on in my body, correct it with wiser food choices, get my body chemistry back on track, and receive normal lab reports at my next yearly physical.

Unbeknownst to me on that day, it would take another 7 1/2 months, due to the Covid pandemic upheavals in the medical business, to find out my cardiovascular and urinary systems were fine. Part of this long wait included a two-month attempt to get an appointment with my favorite nephrologist who would listen to my story and order a 24-hour urine specimen to see if I had high oxalate levels. It took another additional two months to get the 24-hour urine results that revealed my oxalates were moderately high. After seeing the oxalate report, I mentioned to the nephrologist "Imagine how high my oxalate levels would have been had we been able to do the urine test six months earlier when the lab reports revealed those three symptoms." Despite all the long wait and frustration, I was given time to reverse the oxalate toxicity in my body by drinking 12 glasses of water each day for two months to flush out and eliminate the oxalates from all the high oxalate plant foods I had stopped consuming. To this day I am grateful to my nephrologist friend because he told me, "I can't help you because your kidney function is normal." His words gave me hope that I was on the right recovery track. At my recent yearly physical appointment, the 24-hour urine specimen revealed my oxalate levels had returned to the normal range. Once again, I thank you God for your supreme guidance not one of my physicians could offer me.

During this timely research and medical testing process, I am grateful to have been connected to three wonderful oxalate disease preventive professionals. Many thanks to Dr. Michael Liebman, Jill Harris R.N., and Sally K. Norton for educating me about oxalates and their toxicity to the body, a controversial topic with the medical profession. All three of these disease prevention professionals opened my mind to why and how overdoing nutritious plant foods can cause damage to the human body. Jill Harris, RN, offers an oxalate list you may wish to review for more information. To learn more about these foods go to: **https://kidneystonediet.com/oxalate-list/**.

The long months of waiting for the oxalate and cardio stress test results helped me reflect on God's timing for this book. He knew I needed to be humbled to offer my total faith and trust in Him, and to teach us the truth about oxalates, hope, and the patience required for reversing disease.

During this long wait time, God gifted me a spiritual visit I would like to share with you. While preparing for a final cardio stress test that my physician recommended 9 months earlier, I gently slipped into the cardiologist's nuclear stress test machine and laid on my back with my arms reached overhead. I was full of fear and concerned I may have to change the outcome of this book's message to you if the stress test revealed any negative results. At that moment I nervously prayed to God for His will to be done in my life. Then, to calm my body, mind, and spirit, I began a slow deep breathing pattern. Immediately, I felt a spiritual presence gently touch my back as he knelt behind me. His thighs began to support my upper back while his open hands supported my shoulders. Feeling complete peace as I felt his gentle and loving support, I finally trusted whatever the nuclear stress test outcome would be, bad or good. God's will would dictate the completion of this book and the rest of my life.

During this peaceful 30 minutes, as my body was flooded with radiation, a regadenoson injection, and rubidium (a radioactive tracer), the radiologist told me, "You must have a really good insurance company to be paying for this test." Yes, this was a very expensive test.

Before the nuclear stress PET scan test and while an IV was being placed into my right arm, I asked the nurse why I wasn't getting the usual treadmill stress test. She told me the Center for Disease Control and Prevention (CDC) recommended nuclear stress PET scans during the Covid pandemic instead of the regular treadmill stress test and would only allow treadmill tests for special situations. I had no idea about this CDC regulation and was not given a choice by the cardiologist.

Another lesson learned. Ask questions about all recommended tests, and research all medications placed into you before you have them. What I discovered after this test was the radiation that went into my body was 40 times greater than a regular chest X-ray, and the IV medications cause side effects. It scared me when I read that too much radiation can cause cancer.

Once again, as I did with the oxalate toxicity, I flushed my body with extra water for several weeks to help release the harmful effects of the radiation and IVs.

When the nuclear stress test was almost completed, I noticed a nurse had been sitting to my left the entire 30 minutes. Watching her disconnect the blood pressure cuff and IV line, I did notice my heart rate was a good number on the monitor. As I stood up, the radiologist greeted me with a smile and said, "All was fine. Your doctor will call you this evening or tomorrow morning. Did you have any pain in your heart?" Thankfully, I did not have any pain. Unfortunately, the doctor did not call me, as he had stated. Being the proactive patient advocate I am, I allowed the cardiologist 24 hours to call me with the test results. After no phone call, I called the cardiologist's office to get the test results. Sadly, it took a week after the stress test for the cardiologist to contact me with the results. Patience is a virtue but when we are left hanging by a physician's office it can cause unsolicited stress for the patient.

Once again, I understand God answers our prayers with a "Yes," "No," or "Wait." As I have learned, when we wait patiently for His direction, it's much easier when we trust His divine plan for our life 100%. My wellness journey has been filled with new adventures, and I've taken some wrong turns, but I have been graced with determination and perseverance to get myself back on track. As my Godmother Yolie told me years ago, "Pam, sometimes God draws straight with crooked lines." We all have lessons to learn in this life and I wish to share mine with you in hopes that you may bypass them. When you stay true to your goals and keep your heart and mind open, God will lead you to the path of light, for He is our true healer as I witnessed during this entire 9 1/2 month wait time.

As you read about my experiences, if your physician says

that you have some lab report imbalances, be wise and compare your lab reports from the previous year and research what could be the causes for the changes. This will help you decide if you need to change any of your choices or habits. Also, review the last four to six months of your life and make note of what you consumed or what had changed with your choices in food, drinks, supplements, medicines, lotions, environment, relationships, and emotions. Creating a running lab report list for the last two decades has helped me see how my age, lifestyle, and nutrition affect my lab results. Please keep in mind, lab results can be incorrect too. When working in the medical profession and sharing lunch with a physician and his nurse practitioner, I'll never forget him asking his nurse practitioner in front of me, "Are the hospital labs still showing all patient's blood work on the high side?" She responded, "Yes." If you are concerned about faulty lab reports, talk to your physician about it and get retested to gain the complete truth.

PAY ATTENTION TO PORTION SIZES

Ben Franklin, a founding father of the United States who also was a scientist, shared some wellness wisdom we all need to take seriously: "Moderation in all things - including moderation. Eat not to dullness, drink not to elevation."

When you need to change your food choices, it helps to replace unhealthy and highly craved foods with a variety of "moderate" amounts of nutritious foods. Yes, the portion size of what you consume is important in preventing and reversing disease in your body.

There are so many diets out there it can confuse even the best scientist and nutritionist. Becoming aware of the basics of nutrition is important to gaining and maintaining your wellness. Know that our government mandates nutrition for all our physicians, healthcare professionals, and public schools to follow and support their nutrition guidelines. Every five years, the United States Department of Agriculture (USDA) introduces their updated nutrition guidelines called the *Dietary Guidelines for Americans.* The USDA also offers educational websites for consumers and medical/healthcare professionals. To review their nutrition guidelines, go to: **https://www.myplate.gov/**.

Another USDA website you may want to review is https://www.myplate.gov/myplate-plan. As an example, below are the daily amounts of macronutrients and dairy the USDA website prescribed for me according to my age, sex, and activity levels:

Fruits	2 cups
Vegetables	3 cups
Grains	7 ounces
Dairy	3 cups
Protein	6 ounces

I find this interesting. Again, I want to point out there are many nutrition and diet resources that may add confusion to a person trying to figure out what to eat for their best health, weight loss, or vitality. All the nutrition guidance I share with you in this book comes from many reliable resources that helped me reverse the disease in my body. It has been a trial-and-error walk as I discover what works best for my taste buds, energy, health, and happiness. Having yearly physicals with a trusted physician and keeping track of my lab reports is essential for my health accountability.

When you remain focused and mindful about your food choices, you will reach your goals more quickly. If you get off track, return to Chapter 2, "Awareness, The Foundation Of Change," and Chapter 5, "Beginning A Wellness Journey."

Enjoy the portion size visual using my daughter's beautiful hands.

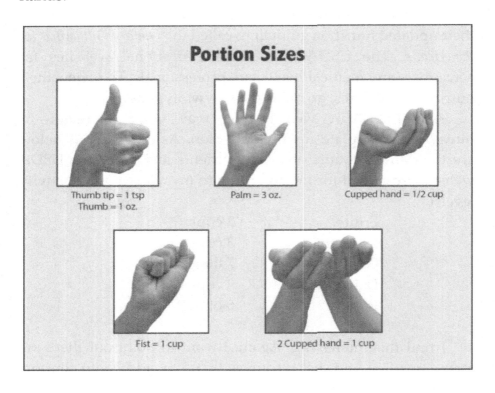

Portion Sizes

Thumb tip = 1 tsp
Thumb = 1 oz.

Palm = 3 oz.

Cupped hand = 1/2 cup

Fist = 1 cup

2 Cupped hand = 1 cup

CHAPTER 9

Sugar Truths And More

Where there is sugar, there are ants.
— Indonesian Proverb

Isn't it amazing how quickly sugary foods and drinks can lift your moods? Dr. Pepper, a Snickers bar, and sometimes two Snickers bars, were my usual pick-me-ups while working in the medical profession for many years. I also loved tasting chewy sweet Bazooka bubble gum and making bubbles while driving around the medical districts. This was a fun habit from childhood. I have no idea how many pieces I chewed each day. My mind was elsewhere.

Why in the world did my mood improve with all the sweet stuff? Many times, it brought back fond memories from my past, just like seeing how big a bubble I could blow with Bazooka bubble gum. Halloween memories were always fun times, and candy certainly was the center of that evening thrill. By the time

I was seven years old, my weekly 25 cents allowance bought many rewarding yummy tastes of Sugar Babies, Sugar Daddies, and Good & Plenty.

Sweet foods can become a comforting ally when our emotions get out of whack. When my dad was on temporary duty for a year, one thousand miles from our home, his favorite ice cream became my food companion. Many people were shocked to see how 30 extra pounds appeared on my 15-year-old frame that year. Think about it: have you ever reached for that special snack, drink, or food, when you need to feel comfort, de-stress, celebrate, or reap rewards for doing a good deed?

While studying to be an Integrative Nutrition Health Coach, my mind was opened wide when I learned how former food choices controlled my brain and entire body. I had no idea processed sweets could activate opiate receptors in my brain and release dopamine every time I ate daily sweets, chewed bubble gum, and drank Dr. Pepper. Even when I thought about them, viewed them, or smelled their sweet aroma, that was enough to release those happy hormones.

All the processed foods I was addicted to contained "added" refined sugars. Never once did it occur to me how sugar was processed until I took time to research it. To my surprise, I learned the United States is among the world's largest sugar producers. I had no idea, that the white sweet granules I used to put on my tongue as a child are extracted from sugarcane and sugar beet crops.[1] During this extraction process, all the plant nutrients are stripped away making refined sugar a "0" nutrient substance. Hmmm? Since sugar has no nutrients, should it be considered a food? Isn't food supposed to nourish and uplift our bodies?

At the beginning of my wellness journey, I began replacing my cravings with nutritious foods. For 38 days, sugar and all foods containing "added" sugar were out of my life! After the initial five weeks of clean eating and new life balance actions, I realized this was an inside-out journey to transform my mind, body, and spiritual fitness. The sugar addiction that once held my health in captivity was released. Feeling positive and energized and walking in the light became a top priority in my life. Gratefully, my former sugar addiction has never returned.

Replacing ice cream, milkshakes, and my favorite Starbucks frozen drinks with a nutritious smoothie helped bust my sugar addiction. Healthy smoothies are an easy, delicious, and fun way to infuse high nutrients and healing energy into your body. The Sugar Busting Smoothie and Wellness Smoothie recipes that helped me bust my cravings are in Chapter 17, "Simple Nutritious Recipes."

More news about the damaging effects of sugar came to me while talking with a nurse. When she heard my desire to help people prevent and reverse disease, she shared a visual lesson a cardiologist once told her. "Pam, when you were a kid, did you ever witness salt being placed on a snail?" I said, "Yes, the poor little snail shriveled up." Then, she said, "Just like that snail, when we consume too much sugar, the same thing happens to our blood vessels. They eventually shrivel up."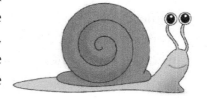

This conversation made me think about the damage sugar was causing within my body and how it helped ruin my father's health. How in the world can sugar do this to our bodies? Think about the 60,000 miles of blood vessels throughout your body. Everything you eat and drink travels from your mouth to your digestive system where it's broken down and transported to your body organs via the blood within your blood vessels.

Have you ever noticed all the Coke and McDonald's billboards along the highways? How about those enticing Starbucks drink pictures smothered in whip cream placed at the front of their doors and drive-thru? Even the fun football game commercials capture our full attention with their alcohol, soda, and food enticements. These subliminal marketing tactics are strategically planned to affect your brain's opiate receptors without you being aware of it. Pretty sneaky, huh? The entire food industry is doing this with all their advertising and product package marketing. So beware, and protect yourself and your family if you want the best energy, health, and happiness.

Before I started my wellness journey, eight extra pounds showed up on the scales during my yearly physical appointment. That afternoon I switched from sweet bubble gum to sugarless bubble gum and from Dr. Pepper to Diet Dr. Pepper. Fewer calories and healthier choices, or at least I thought they were healthier. At that time in my life, I had no idea what controversial ingredients were, nor did I know they were in sugarless gum, diet sodas, and all my favorite processed food choices. No one told me these ingredients could create disease in my body, not even my physician. You will learn more about controversial ingredients in the next chapter, "Clean is Supreme".

SUGAR TRUTHS

When I started my wellness journey and learned that nutritious sugars naturally occur in carbohydrates and milk, this helped me understand that consuming whole foods could enhance my health instead of my junk food choices. This knowledge encouraged me to fuel up on fresh fruits, vegetables, whole grains, and healthy proteins instead of the processed food and drinks packed with added sugars and controversial ingredients, some of the main destructors that affected my body, mind, and spirit.

Do yourself a favor and remember two facts about "added" sugar in processed foods:

- 4 grams of added sugar = 1 tsp of sugar
- White refined sugar has "0" micronutrients

The American Heart Association's (AHA) prevention education helped me understand the main causes of my father's heart disease and why it was happening to me. We both were sugar addicts, professionally stressed, and Type A personalities.

Take a look at AHA's recommended daily "added" sugar amounts per gender and age:

- Men: 9 tsp / 36 grams
- Women: 6 tsp / 24 grams
- Kid's age 2-18:   less than 6 tsp / 24 grams
- Children under 2 should <u>not</u> consume any added sugars[2]

Pleasure seeking, lack of nutrition knowledge, and an unbalanced life blinded my focus on healthy food choices. Never once did I realize a 20-ounce Dr. Pepper is made with 16 teaspoons of added refined sugar. A Snickers bar has 6 ¼ teaspoons of added refined sugar, and one piece of Bazooka Bubble gum has ¾ teaspoon of added refined sugar. I consumed all these products every day and that added up to 23 teaspoons of sugar, 17 more teaspoons than the AHA recommended!

After learning the sugar amounts in these daily junk food choices, I googled the internet for nutrition information after I grabbed containers out of my pantry and refrigerator to read each food label for that day's breakfast, snacks, lunch food, and cough drops. This is what I ate that day: Peach yogurt, low-fat vanilla milk, granola, barbeque sandwich, pork and beans, macaroni and cheese, French fries, ketchup, barbeque sauce, cranberry sauce, Dr. Pepper, Butterfinger, Clif Bar, and Ginger mint cough drops. My eyes popped out of my head when the added amount of sugar reached 76 teaspoons!!! This was 70 more teaspoons than the AHA recommended for women per day.

Has a physician ever told you sugar is the main culprit of heart disease along with many other diseases including diabetes, cancer, thyroid disease, depression, migraines, and 140 more diseases? Dr. Nancy Applegate writes about this in her book, *Lick the Sugar Habit.*

Our brain and stomach take 20 minutes to signal fullness.[3] This time lapse will offer unconscious overeating frenzies as it did for me one afternoon while driving from one client's medical facility to another's. In the back seat of my car sat a basket full of Butterfinger fun-size bars. Looking back at the candy, I thought, "I'll just eat one." By the time I drove into the client's parking lot 10 minutes later, I had devoured 20 fun Butterfinger bars. Talk about a dopamine rush! I had put 40 teaspoons of sugar in my body as my brain receptors screamed for more. This experience was a BIG sugar addiction wake-up call for me.[4]

Too much refined sugar can create weight gain and disease. This is what happened to me! It also affected my moods, energy level, and spirit. I had no idea that too much sugar can:

- Deplete essential vitamins and minerals from the body
- Increase one's appetite stimulation and hunger
- Derail one's appetite for nutrient-dense foods
- Increase bacteria and yeast growth, introducing inflammation into the body[5]

Are you aware of your daily amount of added sugar intake? If not, and if you want to improve your health, begin reading packaged food labels to learn the added amounts of sugar and all the other ingredients. Most popular chain restaurants and fast-food establishments offer food and drink nutrition and ingredient information on their website. It's been a mind opener for me to discover how much sugar, sodium, and controversial ingredients are contained in these foods.

Make time to review the *Micronutrients For Wellness* list in Chapter 8, "Your Food Choices Matter." Reading the body functions for each vitamin and mineral will provide powerful knowledge. You may see correlations in your present health level. If so, this may be the time to begin offering yourself, and the children in your life, whole fresh foods instead of processed foods, candy, cookies, and sugar drinks pumped up with added refined sugar.

To make it through stressful workdays, many of us have suffered from unconscious consumption of fast foods, sweets, sodas, energy drinks, coffee, and tea throughout the day. Never, during one bite, or one sip, did we think our health and peace of mind were being compromised. During this time in my life, pleasure won when it competed with peace.

Do you have a healthy mentor who inspires you? As a young girl, Jack LaLanne, the Godfather of Fitness, intrigued me during his TV shows filled with nutrition, juicing, physical movement, and strengthening education. After busting his sugar addiction, Jack LaLanne created a lifelong wellness journey by balancing his life and eating whole nutritious foods. He inspired many people, including me. Surrounding yourself with healthy people you admire will help you take action and stay motivated. Keep these people and their philosophies close to you at all times. They will help you stay inspired.

Below are the basic goals and actions I used to reverse the disease in my body. All actions began with consistent small steps fueled with determination and perseverance. Each small step helped me conquer that rocky mountain called Sugar Addiction.

- Bust stress
- Defeat sugar addiction
- Remove processed foods out of my life
- Stop eating and driving at the same time
- Sit down and savor every bite while eating

Setting these goals required an honest look at my imbalanced life as well as learning where added refined sugar and energy-depleting ingredients were hiding in the processed foods and drinks I consumed each day. As I discovered, the more knowledge and self-awareness you gain, the more positive actions you will make for the life you want.

WELLNESS GOALS & ACTION TIPS

- Keep daily sugar intake at or below the American Heart Association's recommendations.
- Read the labels and ingredients of all consumed processed food and drinks. This provides you with the

knowledge to try new food adventures and create healthy food substitutes.

- Take time to research unknown food/drink ingredients for any side effects. If it causes side effects, be cautious.
- Look at your favorite restaurant food and drink nutrition information. It will open your mind!
- Be aware of the many different names of sugar hidden in processed foods.

Gaining knowledge about processed food ingredients can help you understand why cravings happen so easily and why the food industry purposely sweetens food. They want your money more than they are concerned about your health or the health of your family.

When you begin reading processed food and drink ingredients you may notice names you have never heard of. Take time to research what they are. See the list below for many sugar names.

DIFFERENT SUGAR NAMES[6]

Agave nectar	Dehydrated cane juice	Maltose
Barbados sugar	Demerara sugar	Maple syrup
Barley malt	Dextrin	Molasses
Barley malt syrup	Dextrose	Muscovado
Beet sugar	Evaporated cane juice	Palm sugar
Brown sugar	Fructose	Panocha
Buttered syrup	Fruit juice/concentrate	Powdered sugar
Cane juice	Glucose	Raw sugar
Cane juice crystals	Glucose solids	Refiner's syrup
Cane sugar	Golden sugar	Rice syrup
Caramel	Golden syrup	Saccharose
Carob syrup	Grape sugar	Sorghum Syrup
Castor sugar	High-Fructose Corn Syrup	Sucrose
Coconut palm sugar	Honey	Sugar (granulated)
Coconut sugar	Icing sugar	Sweet Sorghum
Confectioner's sugar	Invert sugar	Syrup
Corn sweetener	Malt syrup	Treacle
Corn syrup	Maltodextrin	Turbinado sugar
Corn syrup solids	Mannose	Yellow Sugar
Date sugar	Maltol	

Thankfully, in May 2020, the Federal Drug Administration (FDA) required all food manufacturers to list the amount of added sugars in all processed food products. This mandate is to help parents, and all adults, to monitor the daily sugar intake for their children and themselves. Previous to this mandate, none of us knew the amount of added sugar in any processed foods and drinks.

Removing refined sugars from my life became easier when I discovered that sugar has zero micronutrients (vitamins and minerals) and it depleted essential nutrients from my body. I no longer use sugar in my home cooking. I replaced it with nature's real nutritious sweeteners: honey, maple syrup, and molasses. If you are interested in learning the sugar conversion ratio to honey, molasses, or maple syrup for baking and cooking, the internet offers some guidance. Here is a resource I have used for sugar to honey conversion: https://eatbeautiful.net/exact-conversion-chart-sugar-honey-when-baking/.

The sweetness and nutrients in honey are why it's my favorite sugar replacement. Because of its 21 calories and five grams of carbohydrates per teaspoon, I try to limit my daily consumption to three or fewer teaspoons. As with all nutritious foods, moderation is the key.

Take a look at the empowering nutrients in honey, maple syrup, and molasses.

HONEY NUTRIENTS:
Water, B2, B3, B5, B6, B9, Vitamin C, calcium, copper, iron, magnesium, phosphorus, potassium, zinc, selenium, sodium, choline[7.8]

MAPLE SYRUP NUTRIENTS:
Water, B1, B2, B3, iron, calcium, zinc, potassium, magnesium, selenium, phosphorus, sodium, copper, choline[9]

MOLASSES NUTRIENTS:
Water, B1, B3, B6, iron, selenium, magnesium, calcium, sodium, zinc, choline, potassium, phosphorus, copper[10]

SODIUM TRUTHS

Sodium is an electrolyte, a mineral in the body that provides an electric charge. It helps regulate the amount of water in and around your cells. Your body needs a tiny amount of sodium each day to help serve your brain function, blood regulation, fluid balance, nerve impulses, muscle contractions, glucose absorption, blood pressure regulation, muscle cramp prevention, carbon dioxide elimination, and many more essential function processes.[11]

We are all unique individuals, especially in our biology and body chemistry. Sodium requirements differ depending on a person's activity level, age, health condition, and physician guidance. According to the Centers for Disease Control and Prevention (CDC), almost 90% of Americans, 2 years old and older, consume too much sodium, more than double the recommended safe amount.[12]

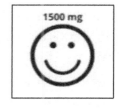

The American Heart Association's (AHA) recommended daily sodium intake for optimal health is no more than 1500 mg. Unfortunately, the average American consumes over 3400 mg, and our children consume over 3100 mg per day, causing an increased risk of high blood pressure, heart attacks, heart failure, stroke, kidney disease, and blindness.[13]

One teaspoon of sodium equals 2300 milligrams (mg), 800 more milligrams than the AHA recommends. If you want to prevent, or reverse disease in your body, pay close attention to the total sodium amounts you and your family consume every day.

The food industry purposely uses sodium to increase taste and visual appeal by enhancing a food's flavor, color, and texture. For example, if you like Chick-Fil-A's chicken sandwich, do yourself a favor and check the sodium amount on their internet nutrition site and all other fast-food establishments you visit. You will notice there are more than 1300 grams of sodium for one Chick-Fil-A chicken sandwich! If you like pizza, one large slice of "The Works" Papa John's Pizza has more than 800 grams of sodium![14] According to the AHA, nearly 80% of a person's sodium consumption comes from their choices of processed food and drinks purchased at grocery stores, fast food drive-thrus, and restaurants. Top sodium enhanced foods include bread, rolls, pizza, sandwiches, cold cuts and cured meats, soup, cheese, chicken, chips, crackers, pretzels, burritos, and tacos.[15]

Did you know that sodium is also used as a preservative to prevent a product from spoiling in a warehouse and sitting on the shelves at the grocery store, restaurant, and in our pantry? Student's eyes bug out when I hold up a five-year-old hamburger bun used in my *Sugar Truth and More* class. The bun, sealed in a plastic baggie, has never molded or spoiled, although it's hard and crunchy now. Like sugar, sodium has many different names. In the following chart, take look at the many sodium names.[16]

Disodium guanylate (GMP)	Sodium citrate
Disodium inosinate (IMP)	Sodium chloride
Fleur de sel	Sodium diacetate
Himalayan pink salt	Sodium erythorbate
Kosher salt	Sodium glutamate
Monosodium glutamate (MSG)	Sodium lactate
	Sodium lauryl Sulfate
Rock salt	Sodium metabisulfite
Salt	Sodium Nitrate
Sea salt	Sodium phosphate
Sodium bicarbonate	Trisodium phosphate

Gaining knowledge about the body's electrolyte balance helped me prepare for a challenging 7-hour Grand Canyon hike from the South Rim to the bottom at Phantom Ranch. Before this challenging hike, I added an ample supply of water, blended with fresh lemon juice and sea salt, to my backpack, along with a nutritious lunch and snacks to provide energy during the hike. The snacks included apples, oranges, beef jerky, and a healthy blend of nuts, seeds, and dried fruit. It was helpful to pack foods that naturally contained electrolytes. Check out the *Micronutrients For Wellness* list in Chapter 8 and see a variety of foods containing electrolytes listed in the sodium, potassium, calcium, phosphorus, and magnesium categories.

WAKE UP AMERICA!

As the adult obesity rates in the U.S. have dramatically climbed to 42.4% and 19. 3% for children age 2 – 19 years old,[17] our government is taking steps to help our country reverse and prevent disease. It would be wonderful if our hospitals did the same. Why does a medical institution that is supposed to prevent harm to their patients have a Starbucks store and vending machines packed with sodas, candy, and high sugar and sodium snacks in their lobbies, gift shops, parking lot area, and cafeterias? Could it be they are promoting sugar and sodium addiction to contribute to their own "Sick Care" income? Several years ago, the local hospitals in my town banned smoking in, or near, their facility. It's time our medical institutions step up to the plate and help their community with food and drink addictions just like they have with smoking addiction.

A couple of years ago, a Kroger manager's wife told me Kroger's biggest selling product was soda drinks. Within a week after hearing this information, the Kroger store near my home remodeled and rearranged all their products. As I walked into the store, I noticed all the soda, chips, crackers, and cookie products were placed near the front and closer to the cash registers. Guess where they used to be? In the back of the store. Have you noticed that most grocery stores place cookies, candy, chips, and sodas in the aisle as you approach the register or in the lobby entrance? The grocery stores know it will set off dopamine in your brain and entice you to purchase more products before you check out. It's time our grocery stores step up to the plate and help heal their community's rising disease levels.

For our community and country to have optimal wellness, it will take all of us holding hands together: individuals, families, community and civic leaders, schools, churches, businesses, physicians, and hospitals. For the future wellness of our children, it is our responsibility to guide them to a lifetime of health, happiness, with lots of joyful energy.

The more positive food choices parents and adults make, the healthier role model they are for the children in their life. Sharing daily clean whole foods during family meals and snack times will empower children to honor and love their precious body, mind, and spirit, their 24/7 home for life.

CHAPTER 10

Clean Is Supreme

Truth is like the sun;
it will rise every day and shine out the darkness.

My head started spinning after hearing all the scary truths at my first class on controversial ingredients, organic and conventional farming, and the pesticides used in farming. Controversial products combined with unconscious eating habits have contributed to the escalating 42.4% adult obesity increases in the United States today. As a result, our children are also experiencing increased obesity and related diseases like never before. The Center for Disease Control and Prevention (CDC) lists the following diseases that are associated with overconsumption of processed food and drinks, a main cause of obesity:

- High blood pressure
- High LDL cholesterol, low HDL cholesterol, or high levels of triglycerides
- Type 2 diabetes
- Coronary heart disease
- Stroke
- Gallbladder disease
- Osteoarthritis
- Sleep apnea and breathing problems
- Many types of cancer
- Low quality of life
- Mental illness such as clinical depression, anxiety, and other mental disorders
- Body pain and difficulty with physical functioning[1]

ALARMING CONTROVERSIAL PRODUCTS AND INGREDIENTS

The emulsifiers, thickeners, artificial sweeteners, and pre-servatives added to processed foods have been reported to have direct and indirect effects on the cells of the body's immune system, contributing to metabolic dysregulation that leads to health imbalances and disease.[2]

When I heard my former physician say, "Pam, you have entered into metabolic syndrome," his words set off a loud alarm that filled my soul with fear and shock. When he asked me, "What is causing all of this?" My quick response was, "Stress from my job!" He then asked, "What are you going to do about it?" What I needed from him was a prescription of hope, resources, and guidance, not another pill to alter the symptoms of my poor food choices, imbalanced life, and stress. Before that day, and more days afterward, I was clueless about harmful food and health-stripping ingredients. How could something so pleasurable hurt me? Like many people today, I was a mummy walking around in the dark and unaware of the truth. It was time to rewire my thinking.

Controversial products are found in the most popular food and drink choices. When these additives and chemicals are regularly consumed, vital nutrients can be depleted, causing many imbalances within our 12 body systems and decreases their ability to properly function. If you have issues with your present health, refer back to the body function column on the *Micronutrients For Wellness* list in Chapter 8 to see what micronutrients your body may be lacking. Self-awareness provides invaluable guidance if you desire change in your life.

The following controversial ingredients education will open your mind to the truth:

PHOSPHORIC ACID

Do you, or a family member, regularly drink sodas? If so, be sure to read this about phosphoric acid that is commonly used to flavor sodas. The use of phosphoric acid remains controversial since it has been associated with adverse health effects. In an article written by Doroto Kregiel, "Health safety of soft drinks: contents, containers, and microorganisms," he states "High levels of phosphorus in the blood, referred to as 'hyperphosphatemia,' can lead to organ damage, most notably of the kidneys. Poor kidney function can raise levels of phosphorus in the blood, which in turn lowers calcium levels, increasing the risk of brittle bone disease. Moreover, increased serum phosphorus levels, as well as other mineral abnormalities, can individually and collectively contribute to vascular calcification and cardiovascular disease."[3] In addition to being used as a flavoring enhancer, it is also used as a non-nutritive sweetener for processed food and drink products. Phosphoric acid is also used as an antimicrobial agent, fumigant, malting or fermenting aid, and a ph control agent.[4]

WHITE SUGAR AND HFCS

Do you have a sweet tooth? Remember there is absolutely no nutritional value to refined sugar because it is stripped of all nutrients during the original plant processing. Sugar and HFCS (high fructose corn syrup) are purposely added in restaurant foods, processed foods, and drinks to enhance their flavor for consumer pleasure. During an Institute of Integrative Nutrition class, one of my instructors, Dr. Mark Hyman stated: "Sugar is eight times more addictive than cocaine." Wow! What a mind opener that was for me! His statement is backed up by a 2007 study in the medical journal, *PLOS One*, titled "Intense Sweetness Surpasses Cocaine Reward."[5] This study concludes that the pleasure of sweet taste outweighs the pleasure from cocaine. HFCS, a liquid sweetener made from corn starch, is much cheaper to produce than regular sugar, so it's used to sweeten sodas, other processed drinks, and food ingredients. HFCS and sugar have been shown to drive body inflammation, which is associated with an increased risk of obesity, diabetes, heart disease, metabolic syndrome, cancer, and many more diseases.[6,7]

ARTIFICIAL SWEETENERS

Artificial sweeteners are chemicals found in more than 6,000 food and drink products. They were introduced into the food industry in World War I and World War II when sugar production was low. These chemicals can sweeten food and drinks 200 to 13,000 times sweeter than white sugar. Just like I used to be, more people are attracted to these products because of their reduced calories and sweetness. Unfortunately, research is discovering that artificial sweeteners are altering insulin sensitivity and creating other disease concerns such as cancer.[8]

At the very beginning of my wellness journey, and before I learned about controversial ingredients, I purchased a box of Klondike *no sugar added* Ice Cream Bars from the grocery store. Nibbling the frozen milk chocolate from the vanilla ice cream was so enjoyable and tasty. Within 30 minutes after my last bite of this frozen pleasure, my mood lowered and my hands started tingling. I quickly read the ingredients on the box and noticed it had aspartame along with many other controversial ingredients. Grabbing my cell phone, I googled aspartame. I learned that dozens of studies have linked aspartame, the world's most widely used artificial sweetener, to serious health problems, including Alzheimer's disease, cancer, cardiovascular disease, stroke, seizures, and dementia, as well as negative effects such as intestinal dysbiosis, mood disorders, headaches, and migraines.[9] Memories of my patients with neurological disorders flooded my soul as I put the remaining ice cream bars in the trash. Never once, since that day, have I ever chosen to eat another food or drink that contained aspartame or other artificial sweeteners.

Learning about the extreme sweetness of artificial chemicals helped me understand how easily my brain and body chemistry were being hijacked when I used to drink Diet Dr. Pepper, chewed sugarless bubble gum, and ate all the "no sugar added" treats. As research continues to reveal the harmful effects of artificial sweeteners, the U.S. Food and Drug Administration (FDA) continues to approve the following chemicals for table sugar replacement to enhance the flavor of processed food and drinks.[10]

Artificial Sweetener	Sweeter Than Sugar
Aspartame	200 times
Acesulfame Potassium (ACE-K)	200 times
Advantame	20,000 times
Luo Han Guo Fruit Extract	100 - 250 times
Neotame	7000 – 13,000 times
Saccharin	200 - 700 times
Sucralose	600 times
Steviol Glycosides	200 - 400 times

If you or anyone in your family experience unusual symptoms in your body, mood, and energy levels, pay close attention to all the ingredients in the processed food and drinks you are consuming. It may be a good time to buy and eat more whole foods if your health and happiness are a priority.

CARRAGEENAN

Meeting with Susan for her health coach sessions was always an honorable time for me because she truly wanted to reverse diabetes and her other health issues. On one particular visit, she slowly slid her revisit form, face down, across the table to me. The revisit form included positive updates from our last session, any new body symptoms, her weight, and the foods she had eaten from our previous session. Looking down the list, I saw diarrhea as a new body symptom. My eyes quickly searched over her food choices. For the first time since we had been working together, I saw that she had eaten ice cream. It had been her birthday, and she wanted to celebrate. "Susan, do you know the brand name of the ice cream you ate?" I asked. When she told me, "Turkey Hill," I asked, "What flavor was it?" "Vanilla," she said with bewilderment. With cell phone in hand, I googled the brand name and ice cream flavor. After reading the ingredients, I handed her my cell phone to read the ingredients. This was a perfect time to explain that her diarrhea side effects were possibly caused by the carrageenan in the ice cream. After that session, I do not recall seeing diarrhea or ice cream on any of Susan's future revisit forms.

Carrageenan, a red seaweed, is used as a thickener, stabilizer, and texturizer in a variety of processed foods and drinks. It can be found in ice cream, dairy products, chocolate milk, coconut milk, soy milk, almond milk, and rice milk. You can also find it in cosmetics, pesticides, pharmaceuticals, toothpaste, and room deodorizers.

Much research is being done to discover the reasons for the U.S. climbing obesity and disease rates in children, teenagers, and adults. One research study revealed inflammatory bowel disease and colorectal malignancy in the United States may be caused by exposure to carrageenan.[11] Another research study states carrageenan may contribute to the development of diabetes and the effects of high-fat consumption.[12] Having personally experienced the side effects of controversial products and witnessing a client who was exposed to carrageenan's side effects opened my mind to heed all these researched warnings.

CAFFEINE

It was news to me when I read that caffeine was the most commonly used drug in the world. "Is caffeine a drug?" I thought. Yes, it is a nervous system stimulant and also a natural ingredient in coffee, teas, and cocoa. It can also be found in medications, supplements, diet pills, sodas, energy drinks, candy, and many processed foods.

An increasing number of clinical studies reveal some caffeine users become highly dependent on caffeine. When people consume too much caffeine for their biochemistry, complications can occur in their cardiovascular and nervous systems. It can also alter a mother's perinatal time frame of birth. Other side effects can include restlessness, nervousness, excitement, insomnia, frequent urination, gastrointestinal disturbance, muscle twitching, tachycardia, arrhythmia, and rambling thoughts or speech.[13]

As the aging process continues, I've noticed drinking one cup of coffee now makes me jittery, so I've checked my blood pressure after drinking a cup, and, to my surprise, it was elevated. Caffeine is absorbed quickly into our body and can be felt within 15 to 30 minutes. It can linger in our body for six hours or longer, reducing our ability to sleep.[14]

Presently, the FDA has cited that "healthy" adults can consume up to a maximum of 400 milligrams of caffeine per day, an equivalent of four or five cups of coffee. Wow! I'd like to see their definition of healthy and the studies verifying this high caffeine amount approval.

Although the FDA has not set a level for children, the American Academy of Pediatrics discourages children and adolescents from consuming any caffeine or other stimulants.[15] Are you aware of all the caffeine sources you consume each day?

If you eat chocolate, drink tea, coffee, sodas, or energy drinks, how do these products affect your mind, body, and spirit? If you want to cut back on your daily caffeine amounts, a good recommendation is to do so gradually. Stopping abruptly may cause withdrawal symptoms such as headaches, anxiety, and nervousness.

MSG (MONOSODIUM GLUTAMATE)

While discussing controversial ingredients at a recent presentation, a young man raised his hand and openly shared his story about having an epileptic seizure after eating food with MSG. When I asked what type of food he was eating, I was surprised that it was Mexican food, not the typical Chinese food we think for MSG.

MSG is one of the most widely used additives in commercial foods to enhance the aroma and flavor. It is placed in canned foods, crackers, meats, salad dressings, frozen dinners, and a myriad of other products found in local supermarkets, restaurants, and school cafeterias. MSG has been linked to behavior changes, obesity, metabolic disorders, headaches, insulin resistance, glucose intolerance, liver damage, Chinese Restaurant Syndrome, neurotoxic effects, and detrimental effects on the reproductive organs.

The FDA is aware of MSG's side effects, although research scientists have not been able to consistently trigger all the reactions to MSG. The FDA considers MSG's addition to processed foods to be "generally recognized as safe."[16]

MSG is the sodium salt of the common amino acid, glutamic acid. It is linked to many other ingredient names as you can see on the next page.[17]

HIDDEN MSG NAMES

Ingredients containing free glutamic acid	Ingredients containing MSG	Ingredients that trigger MSG-toxicity in sensitive individuals
-Glutamic acid (E 620)	-Carrageenan (E 407)	-Corn starch
-Glutamate (E620)	-Bouillon and broth	-Corn syrup
-Monopotassium glutamate (E 622)	-Stock	-Modified food starch
-Calcium glutamate (E 623)	-Flavouring products	-Lipolyzed butter fat
-Monoammonium glutamate (E 624)	-Natural flavour	-Dextrose
-Magnesium glutamate (E 625)	-Maltodextrin	-Rice syrup
-Natrium glutamate	-Oligodextrin	-Brown rice syrup
-Hydrolysed protein	-Citric acid, Citrate (E 330)	-Milk powder
-Calcium caseinate	-Ultra-pasteurized products	-Reduced fat milk
-Sodium caseinate	-Barley malt	(skim; 1 %; 2 %)
-Yeast extract	-Malted barley	-Low fat products
-Torula yeast	-Brewer's yeast	-Vitamin enriched products
-Yeast food	-Pectin (E 440)	-Vinegar
-Yeast nutrient	-Malt extract	-Specific amino acid chelates
-Autolyzed yeast	-Seasonings	such as citrate, aspartate
-Gelatin		and glutamate act as chelat-
-Textured protein		ing agents with minerals
-Whey protein and other related products		supplements
-Soy protein and other products		
-Fortified protein		
-Fermented foods		
-Protease		
-Vetsin		
-Ajinomoto		
-Umami		

E: European numbering system for registered food-additives

Becoming aware of how your body feels after you consume food and drinks is essential to targeting the cause of possible sensitives. Thankfully, the FDA requires foods containing added MSG to be listed in the ingredient panel on the packaging as monosodium glutamate, although, remember there are many other names for glutamic acids and ingredients where MSG is hiding.

Interestingly, MSG naturally occurs in ingredients such as hydrolyzed vegetable protein, autolyzed yeast, hydrolyzed yeast, yeast extract, soy extracts, and protein isolate, as well as in tomatoes and cheeses.

ARTIFICIAL COLORS - DYES

Before entering a wellness journey, it never occurred to me that manufacturers add artificial colors to lure people to buy their products. Little did I know they were made from petroleum, also known as crude oil. These FDA approved artificial dyes are also used in thousands of processed foods and beverages, cosmetics, drugs, supplements, and medical devices.[18]

In 2008 and 2010, the Center for Science in Public Interest (CSPI) petitioned the FDA to ban artificial dyes due to their connection to behavioral problems in children, being a possible carcinogen, causing hypersensitivity reactions, and inadequately tested.[19] Learning these facts about artificial coloring helped me ditch my old addictive junk food habits, some of my cosmetics, and the NyQuil cough syrup that used to sit in my bathroom cabinet.[20,21,22] There is so much to learn for the wanting mind.

SODIUM NITRATE AND NITRITE

Although water and some vegetables such as raw spinach, beets, celery, radishes, and lettuce naturally contain nitrates and sodium, studies reveal that, when added to meat products, this combination potentially forms nitrosamines in the body and increases the risk of cancer. Today, many meat manufacturers add nitrates and sodium during the meat curing process as a preservative, taste and color enhancer, and to prevent microbial contamination and chemical changes. These processed meats include deli meats and cold cuts, ham, bacon, sausages, and hot dogs. When nitrates and nitrites are added to processed meats, studies have found they potentially form nitrosamines in the body which increases the risk of cancer.[23]

The good news is that you can now find nitrate-free meats in most stores. Yesterday, I was at Sprouts and purchased a "Pederson's Natural Farms" Uncured Kielbasa. On the package, it states "NO Nitrate Nitrite Added," "Uncured," "No Sugar," and "MSG Free." It's a blessing to find safe food I enjoy.

ALCOHOL ALERT!

Dr. Libby Weaver, nutritional biochemist and author of *Exhausted to Energized*, wrote "Alcohol is a poison to the human body. It is a poison because we cannot excrete it." A person's liver has to work overtime to turn it into a chemical called acetaldehyde to excrete toxic residue from the body. Alcohol also interferes with the nutritional process of the food and drinks a person consumes by affecting the body's digestion, storage, utilization, and excretion of their nutrients. Excessive and chronic alcohol habits derail the body's fat absorption process, thus impairing the absorption of essential Vitamins A, D, E, and K, and all the B vitamins. It also causes deficiencies in calcium, magnesium, iron, and zinc minerals.[24] Did you know deficiencies of Vitamin A can be associated with night blindness and Vitamin D deficiency is associated with softening of the bones?

In addition to nutritional deficiencies, the CDC (Center of Disease Control and Prevention) reports, that alcohol "can lead to the development of chronic diseases and other serious problems including:

- High blood pressure, heart disease, stroke, liver disease, and digestive problems.
- Cancer of the breast, mouth, throat, esophagus, liver, and colon.
- The weakening of the immune system, increasing the chances of getting sick.
- Learning and memory problems, including dementia and poor school performance.
- Mental health problems, including depression and anxiety.
- Social problems, including lost productivity, family problems, and unemployment.
- Alcohol use disorders, or alcohol dependence."[25]

Dr. Libby Weaver recommends having alcohol-free days in between one 6-oz. consumption of alcohol. The CDC recommends keeping alcohol consumption levels to one 6-oz drink per day for women and no more than two 6-oz. drinks for men. Do you notice the difference between a biochemist's recommendations and our government's recommendations? Which do you choose to follow and why?

Alcohol use continues to be one of the major causes of disease and death in our country. According to the National Highway Safety Traffic (NHST) "Every day, 30 people in the United States die in drunk-driving crashes — that's one person every 50 minutes."[26]

When visiting Kentucky for a Derby Race, a friend offered me some locally made bourbon. Being a nutrition nerd, I looked at the bottle and did not see the usual FDA required ingredients or a food label. Searching the bourbon's website, I did not see any there either. Little did I know the Alcohol and Tobacco Tax Trade Bureau (TTB) of the U.S. Treasury mandates the labeling requirements for all alcohol.[27] It puzzles me as to why most alcohol products are void of any ingredient or nutritional information. Why are they hiding the truth about many alcohol products?

PESTICIDES USED IN U.S. FARMING

I experienced an awakening about the U.S. farming industry while having dinner with a professional chef from a large chicken producer and processing farm. Most of our conversation centered around the food industry. When he told me Roundup® was used on tomato farms, a sudden bolt of lightning ran through my body. I said: "What! You've got to be kidding me?"

Glyphosate, better known as Roundup® (a weed killer) was first registered in 1974 for use in the United States and has been widely used since then to enhance the production of produce. People also apply it in forestry, lawns and gardens, and weeds in industrial areas. According to scientific resources referenced by the National Pesticide Information Center (NPIC), "Glyphosate is an herbicide. It is applied to the leaves of plants to kill both broadleaf plants and grasses. The sodium salt form of glyphosate is used to regulate plant growth and ripen specific crops."[28]

The Monsanto Company initially patented glyphosate and now it is manufactured and sold by many companies and in hundreds of products. Glyphosate has been associated with cancer and other health concerns. As you will read later in this chapter, it is also the herbicide used with "Roundup Ready" genetically modified organisms (GMOs).[29]

So, what are we to do to protect ourselves and our family from this poison used in U.S. food industry production? A helpful produce list for health-conscious consumers is the EWG "Dirty Dozen and Clean 15." This list provides the name of crops sprayed with the most pesticides and the safest conventionally grown produce. Thanks to the Environmental Working Group (EWG), this list is available each year with the latest updates. EWG is a non-profit, non-partisan organization dedicated to protecting human health and the environment. Its mission is to empower people to live healthier lives in a safe environment. With breakthrough research and education, it desires to guide consumer choice and civic action. To learn more about U.S. food and consumer product safety, check out the EWG website: **www.ewg.org.** This is a reliable resource I go to for the latest product research and updates.

ORGANIC VS. CONVENTIONAL FOODS

The mission of the United States Department of Agriculture (USDA) is to feed the United States citizens, to help produce and sell products, not only in our country but around the world. Yes, the USDA desires to feed the world and this means an increase in production which is good for business. The more you sell, the more you have to produce. Hence, the heavy use of pesticides and factory farms in the conventional food market.[30] The increasing awareness of disease prevention has created a large demand for more organically raised foods resulting in an increase of organic farms in the United States. The recent organic farming 2020 survey from the USDA reveals that sales of organic commodities rose by over 31% from 2016 to 2019. Organic farms have increased 17% with the top sales located in California, Washington, Pennsylvania, Oregon, and Texas.[31]

Clients have asked me, "How do you know if food is organic?" My answer: "Look for the USDA organic seal. Organic farms have mandated U.S. Department of Agriculture (USDA) organic standard guidelines they must follow in addition to farm inspections."

The real proof for me has been in taste comparisons and my energy, health, and happiness levels. Eating organically raised foods has been, and still is, nutritious and clean medicine for my body. The produce offers more robust flavors than the blah-tasting conventional ones. Grapes, strawberries, red peppers, and sweet potatoes are excellent examples if you want to try a taste comparison between organic and conventionally grown produce. During a recent card game gathering, one of my friends was eating the organic vegetables and hummus I placed on the table. She said, "Wow, Pam, these red peppers are so delicious!" That was a cue to let my friends know all the vegetables on the plate were organic. I also said, "Organic produce is not only healthier, but it is also tastier than conventional food, as you just experienced."

One of my clients happened to be there and confirmed what

I said about the taste. If the cost of organic food concerns you, there is good news! Not all produce has to be organic for disease prevention unless you choose so. Having a copy of the EWG's "Dirty Dozen and Clean 15" produce list, or cell phone downloaded copy, is helpful when shopping for produce at the grocery store. It's helpful to know what produce has large amounts of pesticides and which ones do not.

Four food categories qualify as USDA organic standards: Crops—Livestock—Wild crops—Processed / Multi-Ingredient Products. All this food must be 100% organically grown or, if processed, the processed food product must have at least 95% organic ingredients. The methods and standards used in growing or raising farmed food are the main differences between organic and conventional foods. Per the USDA, "All organic products must be protected from prohibited substances and methods from the field to the point of final sale, whether it is a raw agricultural commodity or a multi-ingredient, processed product."[32]

USDA labeled organic crops and livestock must be raised in a production system that emphasizes:

- Protection of natural resources, plant, and animal health.
- Preventative management of pests, diseases, and predators.
- Compliant use of allowed materials.

Organic operations must maintain or enhance soil and water quality while also conserving wetlands, woodlands, and wildlife. Synthetic fertilizers, sewage sludge, irradiation, and genetic engineering may not be used.

Digging a little deeper into our country's farm production

processes, the Organic Trade Association (OTA) reveals more differences between organic and conventional farming methods. In the past, organic farmers had restricted access to 27 synthetic active pest control products while conventional farming had more than 900+ registered synthetic active pest control products. OTA also reported organic ranchers had restricted access to 37 synthetic livestock health treatments, while more than 550 synthetic active ingredients are approved in conventional animal drug products.[33] These products and numbers have changed as time and research have moved forward. The good news is that before organic farmers can use any synthetic active pest control products, they must try all mechanical, cultural, biological, and natural materials first. If you are interested in learning more about the U.S. organic regulations google **The National Organic Program: USDA Organic Regulations.** This site provides a document announcing the renewal of substances listed on the National List of Allowed and Prohibited Substances within the U.S. Department of Agriculture's (USDA) organic regulations.

The most alarming information I've learned about U.S. livestock, is that 80% of all antibiotics sold in the U.S. have been prophylactically used for animals raised in factory farms. This information was shared by another wonderful instructor, Mark Bitman, when I attended the Institute of Integrative Nutrition. Mark Bitman is an author, speaker, and Special Advisor on Food Policy at Columbia University's Mailman School of Public Health.

Do yourself a favor and make time to watch a Factory Farm YouTube video to learn how our country's major meat supply is produced. You will see animals in constant compressed living conditions, unable to roam and graze on grass farms, and restricted from breathing fresh air. The heavy antibiotic injection use in factory-farmed animals helps prevent the spread of animal infections. Unfortunately, these injections can cause health threats to any consumer by inadvertently promoting the spread of antibiotic-resistant strains of bacteria into their body.

Do you prefer your meals made by a person who prepared whole clean food with love in their heart, or meals created in a factory, in a fast-food production line, or a highly processed food injected with toxic antibiotics and chemicals?

One thing we all must remember is that what goes into the food we eat, including how it is treated with either loving care or abuse, and how it is prepared, with love or factory processing, flows into our bodies. Every time you eat or drink, your choices affect you, either positively or negatively.

During a private grocery store class with my client Renae, I asked her to point out a healthy food she enjoys and we would compare the cost and nutrition value to the organic red pepper I showed her in the produce department. Renae went straight to the bakery department and picked up a box of blueberry muffins. After she read the muffin ingredients she looked at me like a deer in headlights and said, "You got me on that one, Pam. I AM addicted to sugar." Renae quickly learned about health destructive cravings versus the value of enriching nutrition.

For more organic and conventional farming education and their latest updates, google the USDA and the OTA websites and key in your questions.

DAIRY, MEATS, EGGS, and SEAFOOD

Before attending the Institute of Integrative Nutrition, I had no clue what was going on in the U.S. dairy, meat, seafood, and egg production industries and how these products evolved to grocery stores, fast-food establishments, and restaurants. Thankfully, my mind was opened and the truth helped me make healthier choices.

Regarding the USDA organic standards, there are some differences and similar regulations for dairy, meat, eggs, and seafood. Each is grown in its unique environmental settings and processed differently.[34]

As always, when you grocery shop, read the food labels. Any added ingredients on the product package are important for you to know. Try not to be swayed by all the marketing tactics used on the product packaging. For example, the FDA defines the word "natural" as nothing artificial or synthetic (including all color additives regardless of source) has been included in, or has been added to, a food that would not normally be expected to be in that food.[35] However, this policy was not intended to address food production methods, such as the use of pesticides, nor did it explicitly address food processing or manufacturing methods, such as thermal technologies, pasteurization, or irradiation. To choose a safer food choice, I look for the USDA Organic label on the product packaging.

DAIRY

As you will read later on in this chapter, milk is the number one food allergen in the United States. Could this be pointing to conventional milk, rather than organic milk? Milk is also shown to be the main drink on the USDA Food Plate. Why is milk the featured drink on the USDA Food Plate and not water? Water is essential to life and maintains our overall health and well-being. Do you think the USDA could be marketing for the dairy farmers on the USDA Food Plate instead of thinking about the health of its country?

For a cow's milk to be labeled by USDA organic standards, each cow must get plenty of fresh grass and spend at least four months a year grazing in pastures. They are to be fed organic food with no Genetically Modified Organisms (GMOs) or given any antibiotics or added hormones. Cheese, yogurt, butter, ice cream, whey, and milk powder are all products of milk. Consider how the cow was raised and fed if you desire an organic or conventional dairy product.

MEAT

The marketing words on meat and poultry packages can be confusing. To learn more about the meat and poultry labels and what they mean, google USDA and search "Meat and Poultry Labeling Terms." There you will see definitions such as certified, chemical-free, fresh poultry, and free-range. Did you know "fresh poultry" means the whole poultry and the cut pieces have never been below 26 degrees?[36] Learning this scared me so I have taken time to seek the truth for all USDA and FDA food definitions.

EGGS

With so many different choices in the egg department, most people go for the cheaper dozen unless they know how the hens were raised and fed. Generally, you think "cage-free" means chickens can freely roam on pasture land. The USDA states cage-free eggs are produced by hens housed in a building, room, or enclosed area that allows for unlimited access to food and water and provides the freedom to roam within the area during the laying cycle. All my students and clients are shocked to learn cage-free chickens are not allowed to roam outside.[37] I personally purchase organic pasture raised eggs.

SEAFOOD

If you enjoy seafood, open your mind to this education. The National Oceanic and Atmospheric Administration U.S. Department of Commerce (NOAA) and NOAA's FISHWATCH are the leading science authorities for managing the U.S. marine fisheries. The U.S. government agency, FISHWATCH, is responsible for monitoring and enforcing marine fisheries within 4.4 million square miles and 95,000 coastland miles of the U.S. exclusive economic zone. There are two types of commercial seafood to choose from, wild and farmed fish. Over the last 30 years, wild-capture fisheries have not been able to meet the increasing domestic demand, so aquaculture (farmed fish) has increased to help supply this demand. Aquaculture farming has become the world's fastest growing form of food production.[38] The United States produces a relatively small amount of seafood from aquaculture and relies heavily on foreign aquaculture imports to meet the growing demand for healthy protein, omega fatty acids, vitamins, and minerals that benefit the heart, brain, and entire body.

Aquaculture is the breeding, rearing, and harvesting of fish, shellfish, algae, and other organisms in all types of water environments. The U.S. freshwater aquaculture produces species native to its rivers, lakes, and streams. Catfish is the top-produced fish, followed by trout, tilapia, and bass. Approximately half the seafood eaten worldwide, including in the United States, is now farm-raised.[39]

NOAA estimates the United States imports more than 80 percent of the seafood from China, Thailand, Canada, Indonesia, Vietnam, and Ecuador. A significant portion of this imported seafood is actually caught by American fishermen, exported overseas for processing, and then reimported to the United

States. The top U.S. imports (by volume) include shrimp, freshwater fish, tuna, salmon, groundfish, crab, and squid. All seafood sold in the United States is required to have the country of origin label on the package.[40]

The largest single sector of U.S. marine aquaculture is oysters, clams, mussels, shrimp, and salmon. Seaweed is also grown for food, medicine, and other uses. Marine Aquaculture can take place in the ocean (in cages on the seafloor or suspended in the water column) or on land in enclosed systems.

Freshwater aquaculture occurs in ponds and on land with enclosed systems producing catfish, trout, tilapia, and bass. The U.S. seafood farmers follow the same food safety guidelines as all other livestock farmers. Vaccines are used to prevent disease in farmed fish along with the use of antibiotics and other drugs. A farmer may, in consultation with a licensed veterinarian, use a limited number of aquatic animal drugs when approved by the FDA to treat specific conditions.

If you would like to learn more about seafood sold in the U.S., google FishWatch.gov or NOAA.gov to get more facts about U.S. seafood harvesting. Seafoodwatch.com is another resource I use to gain information about responsible seafood choices in my location.

WHAT IS GMO?

In the 1990s, the first Genetically Modified Organisms (GMO) crops entered the U.S. food industry. Genetic modification is a special set of gene technology that alters the genetic mechanism of plants, animals, and organisms. Like all new technologies, some risks are created, both known and unknown. Controversies and public concerns surrounding GMO foods and crops commonly focus on human and environmental safety.

143

Herbicide tolerance is the most prevalent GMO trait engineered into food crops. Glyphosate is best known as the active ingredient in Roundup-branded herbicides, and the herbicide used with "Roundup Ready" GMOs.[41] As GMO seeds mature into a plant, they are also able to withstand toxic pesticide spray. Remember, what goes in a GMO produced plant, goes into your body when you consume it.

Approximately 90% of our supermarket food is conventionally grown using GMO seeds. Health risks associated with GMO foods are concerned with toxins, allergens, or genetic hazards.[42]

Here are the top U.S. GMO crops:

Soy
Corn
Canola
Cotton
Zucchini
Sugar Beets
Yellow Squash
Hawaiian Papaya

GMO plants are major ingredients for most of the processed food and drinks you purchase at grocery stores, food establishments, and restaurants. Popular products and food ingredients derived from these crops include oils, soy protein, soy lecithin, cornstarch, granulated sugar, corn syrup, and high fructose corn syrup. More than 95% of animals used for meat and dairy in the United States are fed from GMO crops. Organic regulations prohibit organically raised livestock to be fed GMO feed.[43] Unless you see the USDA organic seal or Non-GMO wording, the ingredients are made with GMO products.

When I learned about GMOs, once again, I was inspired to purchase more organic foods and increase homemade meals.

TOP U.S. FOOD ALLERGENS

When I first learned about the top food allergens, I began a two-week elimination of all dairy, eggs, and wheat to see if my energy, digestion, and moods would change. Luckily, all was fine when I reintroduced these particular foods back into my life, one at a time. Intentionally, each food I reintroduced was organically grown.

According to the Federal Department of Agriculture (FDA), more than 160 foods cause allergic reactions in humans, although 90 percent of allergic food reactions are caused by these nine foods:[44]

1. Milk
2. Eggs
3. Fish (bass, flounder, cod)
4. Crustacean shellfish (crab, lobster, shrimp)
5. Tree nuts (almonds, walnuts, pecans)
6. Peanuts
7. Wheat
8. Soybeans
9. Sesame

If you happen to be sensitive to any of these foods, consider how they were raised or farmed. Were they filled with pesticides, antibiotics, or other health damaging ingredients?

Food allergies may cause havoc in your body within an hour after consumption if you are allergic to the food. Symptoms may range from sneezing to a sudden rash or hives, nasal congestion, swollen lips or other swollen body parts, indigestion, and dizziness. In severe cases, swelling of the throat, irregular heartbeats, shock, and unconsciousness may happen. Seek medical help right away if you experience any of these symptoms.

Most of us are not focused on how we feel right after we eat unless we have a severe reaction. If you want to become more in tune with your body, pay attention to how you feel after you eat. If you begin to feel a sudden change in your energy level or have side effects or symptoms, I recommend eliminating all suspicious foods for two weeks to see if you start to feel more energy, fewer aches and pains, and improved overall wellness. Keeping a daily food diary and documenting how you feel after each meal during this two-week elimination time will increase your awareness and help you pinpoint foods or drinks you may be sensitive to. If you wish to re-introduce eliminated food back to your daily choices, slowly add back one item at a time for two weeks to see if you have any reactions. This was a valuable method for me when I reintroduced organic dairy, eggs, and wheat products back into my food choices instead of the conventional farmed product.

BE SMART: READ ALL FOOD LABELS & INGREDIENTS

In 2020, the FDA mandated Nutrition Facts labels on all processed food and drink packaging to reflect new scientific information, including the link between diet and chronic diseases such as obesity and heart disease. (This does not include alcohol products.) The new food label was created for consumers to have more information to make healthier food choices. The FDA began by announcing that new label changes were coming in May 2016,[45] although food manufactures were given until May 2020 to comply with the new food label mandates. Change can be a slow process, even for our government.

Below are two generic food label samples. Note the new label on the right reveals a larger print for the calories for a 2/3 cup serving size, *added* sugar, and the percent Daily Value (%DV) shows how much macronutrient and some micronutrients in a serving size.

Nutrition Facts		
Serving Size 2/3 cup (55g)		
Servings Per Container About 8		
Amount Per Serving		
Calories 230	Calories from Fat 72	
		% Daily Value*
Total Fat 8g		12%
Saturated Fat 1g		5%
Trans Fat 0g		
Cholesterol 0mg		0%
Sodium 160mg		7%
Total Carbohydrate 37g		12%
Dietary Fiber 4g		16%
Sugars 1g		
Protein 3g		
Vitamin A		10%
Vitamin C		8%
Calcium		20%
Iron		45%

* Percent Daily Values are based on a 2,000 calorie diet. Your daily value may be higher or lower depending on your calorie needs.

	Calories:	2,000	2,500
Total Fat	Less than	65g	80g
Sat Fat	Less than	20g	25g
Cholesterol	Less than	300mg	300mg
Sodium	Less than	2,400mg	2,400mg
Total Carbohydrate		300g	375g
Dietary Fiber		25g	30g

Nutrition Facts	
8 servings per container	
Serving size	**2/3 cup (55g)**
Amount per serving	
Calories	**230**
	% Daily Value*
Total Fat 8g	10%
Saturated Fat 1g	5%
Trans Fat 0g	
Cholesterol 0mg	0%
Sodium 160mg	7%
Total Carbohydrate 37g	13%
Dietary Fiber 4g	14%
Total Sugars 12g	
Includes 10g Added Sugars	20%
Protein 3g	
Vitamin D 2mcg	10%
Calcium 260mg	20%
Iron 8mg	15%
Potassium 235mg	6%

* The % Daily Value (DV) tells you how much a nutrient in a serving of food contributes to a daily diet. 2,000 calories a day is used for general nutrition advice.

This is wonderful information for the United States consumers because no one ever knew the amount of added sugar to any products before the recent 2020 label.

The FDA states it is now rare that people are deficient in Vitamins A and C, although Vitamin D and potassium have taken their place on the new label as more deficiencies occur in these essential micronutrients.

When you read ingredients on packaged and canned foods, know they are listed in descending order of predominance by weight. This means the ingredient that weighs the most is listed first and the ingredient that weighs the least is listed last.

This ingredient list came from an eight-year-old macaroni and cheese box used in many *Sugar Truths and More!* workshops. Do you know why vitamins were added to this product and what all the ingredients are? Because nutrients are destroyed during whole grain processing, the FDA mandates food fortification for processed foods to provide supplemented nutrients to replace the real ones that were destroyed.[46]

INGREDIENTS: ENRICHED MACARONI PRODUCT (WHEAT FLOUR, NIACIN, FERROUS SULFATE [IRON], THIAMIN MONONITRATE [VITAMIN B1], RIBOFLAVIN [VITAMIN B2], FOLIC ACID); CHEESE BLEND (WHEY, MODIFIED FOOD STARCH, SALT, MILKFAT, MILK PROTEIN CONCENTRATE, CONTAINS LESS THAN 2% OF SODIUM TRIPOLYPHOSPHATE, CELLULOSE GEL, CELLULOSE GUM, CITRIC ACID, SODIUM PHOSPHATE, CALCIUM PHOSPHATE, LACTIC ACID, YELLOW 5, YELLOW 6, ENZYMES, CHEESE CULTURE).

CONTAINS: WHEAT, MILK.

Take a moment to reflect on your primary goals. If one of your goals is to prevent or reverse disease, examining the quality of all things you put in your body is essential. Your transformation will happen when you renew your mind with educational truths, consume more clean whole foods, and balance your life.

In Chapter 11, "How Your Body Communicates To You," you will learn how your body speaks when you are experiencing discomfort and pain. When this happens, it would be wise to review all the processed food and drinks you consumed by reading the food label and ingredient list. Be sure to search any fast food and restaurant websites, or ask the manager for the ingredients in the food you eat from these establishments. From personal experience, I have learned the food I choose can be my best medicine or my slowest poison.

CHAPTER 11

How Your Body Communicates To You

If you listen to your body when it whispers,
you won't have to listen to it when it screams.

Chad was an intelligent and happy 3-year-old boy whom I met one morning at Starbucks. His mom brought him along to our first business meeting. When buying her coffee, she also bought Chad a piece of Starbuck's pumpkin bread. When Chad finished his treat, within minutes he turned into a complaining, crying, cranky little boy saying, "I want another piece of pumpkin bread!" Pulling out my cell phone to research the pumpkin bread ingredients, I read that it had 10 teaspoons of added sugar! While sharing this news with his mom, she knew about dopamine release and how quickly it caused a negative biochemical response to his brain, body, and mood changes. Chad and his mom were blessed by this scary yet valuable lesson. From that day forward, she has paid close attention to the food she gives her son to prevent disease from entering his life.

What goes in, around, and what touches you, affects your entire body, mind, and spirit. Your body uses simple messages when it communicates. No words, just feelings and reactions to your daily choices, your lifestyle, and your environmental surroundings. Receiving communication from your body can happen through your energy levels, your moods, emotions, pain, and other physical signs. For optimal wellness, the key to listening to your body is to become aware of any unconscious and conscious cravings, perceptions, thoughts, and habits.

It's interesting to learn how all your body's organs and systems work in unison to communicate a message to you. For example, your Enteric Nervous System (ENS) is very sensitive to stress and emotions. Your ENS is also known as your second brain, gut, or gastrointestinal tract and is capable of working independently of your central nervous system that includes your brain and spinal cord.[1] Your Celiac Plexus, better known as Solar Plexus, is located near your ENS, stomach, and aorta. It's a large cluster of nerves that relay messages from the major organs of your abdomen to your brain. Your heart, responsible for pumping oxygenated and nutritious blood throughout your entire body, also expresses deep emotional feelings. Imagine them all positioned close together working in unison with your entire digestive system, nervous system, and brain. When you receive a "gut feeling," think of it as a unified communication for you to open your mind and listen. When you pay attention and follow what your gut says to you, this will help you detour many hard lessons in life.

Your body also speaks loud and clear to you when it experiences negativity in any form. Symptoms may include pain, low energy, indigestion, constipation, diarrhea, bowel changes, headaches, thinning hair, brittle nails, hormonal changes, depression, hyperactivity and other mental health issues, slow healing, confusion, and lack of concentration.[2]

Paying attention to any negative body response within minutes to 24 hours after they appear can open your mind to the cause-and-effect concept. When negative symptoms occur, ask yourself these questions:

- What did I do within the last 24 hours?
- How is my daily hydration?
- Did I try a new food or drink?
- Did I eat at a new restaurant?
- Did I begin a new medication, supplement, lotion, or treatment of any kind?
- What environments was I exposed to?
- Who did I speak to and share time with?
- Were there any negative emotions or sensations during this time frame?
- How much TV, internet, social media, and gaming am I doing each day, and when?
- How are my sleep patterns? Am I getting enough sleep?
- Do I have stress? If so, what is causing it?

Your answers may help reveal the cause of any pain, discomfort, or negative symptoms. Once you discover the cause, you can work to eliminate, reduce, or adapt it. Keeping a daily journal of how you feel each day is beneficial. If your symptoms persist, you may want to seek guidance from a trusted physician, counselor, therapist, or health coach.

An imbalanced circadian rhythm, your sleep and wake cycle, can be another reason your body may send you subtle communication. According to the Sleep Foundation, "Your circadian rhythm is basically a 24-hour internal clock that is running in the background of your brain and cycles between sleepiness and alertness at regular intervals. It's also known as your sleep/wake cycle." Most humans experience a natural drop in energy between 1:00 pm and 3:00 pm.[3] Before my wellness journey, I was not aware of this mid-day energy slump or what caused it. For years, I would infuse my body with sweet snacks and caffeine drinks to energize me during the middle of the day. Little did I know that these choices robbed my body of essential nutrients and contributed to my body dysfunctions and disease.

If regular midafternoon hunger happens, addressing it with clean whole foods is the way to go. A valuable lesson I learned was to take a break, drink some water, and eat a nutritious snack. A few mid-afternoon snacks I choose include a piece of fresh or frozen fruit topped with organic Greek yogurt and a few nuts or seeds. I also enjoy some hummus and fresh vegetables with half a sandwich. This helps curb hunger and infuses my body with healthy nutrients and sustainable energy.

Listen to your body. It speaks to you all the time when it's happy, sad, or not feeling well. Responding to its compassionate communication will help you set healthier boundaries if your body, mind, and spirit have weakened.

CHAPTER 12

Setting Healthy Boundaries

Self-love, self-respect and self-awareness are protective barriers.

Envision a wooden fence next to a beautiful field of green grass, flowers, songbirds, abundant nature, and sunshine. On the other side of the fence is a field of weeds, rocks, mosquitos, ticks, lizards, and snakes. Which side of the fence would you prefer to live on?

If you chose the beautiful side, your spirit would most likely be lifted with abundant peace, joy, and love each day. Do you think the mosquitos, ticks, lizards, and snakes would honor and respect the fence boundary and not enter the other side?

Each of us is like this beautiful garden, open to everything around us. Fences can be crossed by anything and anyone. Learning to say NO to harmful lifestyle choices, negative people, time zappers, mindless habits, and energy depleters is a powerful step to protect your energy, health, and happiness.

If you are a person who puts others' needs before yours, Dr. Henry Cloud and Dr. John Townsend, have valuable guidance for you in their many books, especially *Boundaries* and *Safe People*.

Many of my clients receive a copy of *Boundaries* to help them learn about themselves and gain strength in saying "NO" to things that zap their life.

Setting boundaries can be formed in different ways. Below are some examples for finding more peace in your life:

- **Physical Boundaries** help you determine who may touch you, your property, and under what circumstances.
- **Mental Boundaries** give you the freedom to safeguard your thoughts and opinions.
- **Emotional Boundaries** help you deal with your own emotions and disengage from any harmful, manipulative, or controlling emotions of others.
- **Spiritual Boundaries** offer you the freedom to deepen your relationship with God or your divine entity.

If you seem to run out of personal time every day, go back to Chapter 5, "Beginning a Wellness Journey," and review the clock tool to see where you are spending your time. Review what you value in life and what your top priorities are.

Is it time to set some boundaries and stick to them? You deserve to be respected and honored in all ways, and by everyone, including yourself.

CHAPTER 13

Healing Sleep

Sleep is essential for wellness. It releases debris from your day and allows healing to take place.

Mrs. Jenkins' anger exploded as I walked into her private nursing home room at 8:00 a.m. We had a date to start her first Occupational Therapy (OT) treatment after a recent hip replacement surgery that left her immobile. The plan was to practice safe transfers from her bed to a wheelchair and to use a walker for safe mobility. After my good morning greeting, her first words were: "I called the police earlier this morning. No one would come and help me to the bathroom after I pressed the nurse call button several times." After allowing her time to release her anger and settle down, I asked her how long she had waited for the nursing staff before she called the police. "Thirty minutes!" she said. The police alerted the administrative office and help came to her right away. Amazed by her actions, I decided bowel and bladder education would be a part of our OT session. Imagine how it must feel to need to go to the bathroom if you are not able to get up on your own. Her guidance included the following bowel and bladder tips:

- Abstain from fluid consumption several hours before bedtime which will decrease the need to urinate during sleep.
- Plan a bathroom visit every two hours, each day and evening, to help condition your body and sensation awareness.
- Make one last bathroom trip before you turn off your lights at night.

One more tip I gave her was: "Hit your nurse call button when you feel the slightest urge to go to the bathroom. The nursing staff is constantly helping other patients who also need to go to the restroom." Thankfully, this situation never happened again.

I'm amazed how many clients suffer poor sleep due to their full or aging bladders waking them up in the middle of their sleep. Quality sleep is a premier prescription for health. It helps with weight management, mental focus, physical performance, energy and mood levels, and it rejuvenates your skin.

Sleep offers your body healing time as your brain goes into recharge mode. Any built-up physical, emotional, and mental stress from your day is released during sleep. When your sleep is constantly interrupted, any built-up debris from the day will compound, and more cortisol will flood into your body, compromising your entire being.

Before starting a wellness journey, quality sleep was not a part of my life and contributed to all my health breakdowns.

According to the Centers for Disease (CDC), insufficient sleep has been linked to the development of chronic diseases and conditions, including Type 2 Diabetes, cardiovascular disease, obesity, and depression.

How does this happen? Insufficient sleep affects your growth hormone secretion linked to obesity. As the amount of hormone secretion decreases from loss of sleep, the chance of weight gain increases. Your blood pressure usually falls during sleep; however, interrupted sleep can adversely affect this normal decline, leading to hypertension and cardiovascular problems. Research has also shown that insufficient sleep impairs the body's ability to use insulin, which can lead to the onset of diabetes.

While sleep disturbance has been a symptom of depression, recent research has indicated that depressive symptoms may decrease if sleep apnea has been diagnosed, effectively treated, and sufficient sleep is restored.[1,2] It could be time for a sleep study if you are suffering from depression.

An average of 7-9 hours of quality sleep is recommended for most adults.[3] Sleeping without an alarm clock is a good method to discover how much sleep your body needs. When I tried this, my body consistently communicated it needed 9 hours for peak performance. If you have sleep issues, below are three important questions to answer:

1. What over stimulates me?
2. What soothes my body, mind, and spirit?
3. How do I feel when I wake up each morning?

What overstimulates you may prevent quality sleep. What soothes you may provide better sleep. How you feel before you go to bed or wake up each morning can reveal what is good for you and what is not. Being conscious of your choices and how they make you feel is a big self-awareness step. Remember, you can only heal what you feel and reveal.

MAJOR SLEEP DISRUPTORS

Eating stuffed jalapeno peppers at dinner taught me a valuable lesson. After tossing and turning in bed for four hours, it finally dawned on me that spicy food prevented me from having a good night's sleep. At that time, I had no idea capsaicin, a component in spicy peppers can increase a person's body temperature and energy levels, causing a reaction known as thermogenesis.[4] As I learned the hard way, if consuming spicy foods affects your sleep, it's best to enjoy them during breakfast or lunchtime, instead of dinner.

Reflect on these questions if you experience negative sensations in your body. All these factors may affect your quality of sleep for better or worse.

- How do I feel after a meal, a snack, and any consumed fluids?
- How do I feel after taking any medications, supplements, or over-the-counter drugs?
- How do I feel after watching TV, working on the computer, gaming, or scanning through my cell phone?
- How do I feel after an evening walk in the fresh air and spending time in nature?
- How do I feel after reading a simple book before bedtime?

- Does my bedroom offer darkness, quiet, coolness, and peace to help induce quality sleep?
- Do I lie awake at night thinking or worrying? If so, what calming or spiritual practices can help me release these thoughts and worries?
- If you have a pet(s), are they on your sleep schedule? Are they sleeping in a comfortable area with a proper temperature for their body?

The pineal gland located in your brain is responsible for the secretion and release of melatonin, a sleep-inducing hormone. Melatonin is regulated by your circadian rhythm and suppressed by light stimuli. Darkness stimulates the release of melatonin.[5] When you use a television, computer, or cell phone before bedtime it may shut off your melatonin production. Avoiding screen devices one to two hours before bedtime is a good habit to ensure restful sleep.

ALCOHOL CONSUMPTION

A small glass of wine may not cause much harm unless that one glass turns into two, three, four, or five glasses a night, many times a week. Partaking in several alcoholic drinks before bedtime causes your digestive system, including your liver and kidneys, to work overtime to process the alcohol out of your body. This processing can cause many people to wake at 2:00 a.m. Since alcohol depletes essential nutrients from the body, the next day most people feel a decrease in their energy, unaware of the cause. Does this happen to you?

Reducing alcohol consumption may take us outside of our comfort zone at first, but in time it will help us to grow, change, and transform our life. Some people drink more alcohol when they are stressed, suffering from emotional imbalances, or just want to socialize and have fun with others. Some alternatives to drinking alcohol can include:

- Enjoy quality time with friends and family.
- Incorporate daily relaxation techniques.
- Spend more time in nature.
- Activate joyful physical movement each day.
- Create and maintain a spiritual life.

MEDICAL CONDITIONS

According to the Sleep Foundation Organization, some medical conditions can compromise sleep such as:

- Thyroid imbalances
- Restless leg syndrome
- Chronic pain issues
- Chronic gastro problems
- Snoring and sleep apnea
- Depression, high levels of stress, anxiety, and fear

These medical situations have a strong possibility of improving when a person becomes aware of their unconscious habits, makes healthier food and drink choices, and balances their life.[6]

REGULATING YOUR CIRCADIAN RHYTHM

Have you observed nature's rhythm? Most birds and animals go to sleep when it gets dark and awaken in the morning's light. Like nature, having a ritual bedtime and wake-up time will help provide you a balanced circadian rhythm, quality sleep, and better health.

Your circadian rhythm is a 24-hour internal clock that's regulated by several hormones and cycles that range between sleepiness and alertness at regular intervals.[7] Did you know hormones are partially regulated by your food choices and physical movement? Physical movement on a regular schedule can help normalize your circadian rhythm and induce quality sleep.

SLEEP INDUCING FOODS

Whole foods, in moderation, can be a healthier alternative to a sleeping supplement or pill laden with negative side effects. Adding sleep-inducing foods into your last meal, or an evening snack, at least two to four hours before bedtime, will help stimulate the release of serotonin, a neurotransmitter that calms your brain for better sleep. Complex carbohydrates and foods containing tryptophan, melatonin, and phytonutrients are linked to improved sleep outcomes.[8,9] Some foods that may improve sleep include:

- Tart cherries, Dark grapes, Strawberries, Bananas
- Legumes, Nuts, Seeds (sesame and pumpkin/pepitas)
- Oats, Rice, Barley
- Milk, Eggs, Fish, Mushrooms

PRE-BEDTIME SOOTHING TIPS

Creating a calm foundation of peace, contentment, and gratefulness before bedtime will enhance your quality of sleep. Below are some of the things I do. Try them all to discover the ones that work best for you.

- Soaking in a warm bath scented with lavender essential oil.
- Gentle floor stretches or using a foam roller to release any tightness in the neck, shoulders, hips, and back.
- Listening to soft relaxing music.
- Reading a book that requires soul thinking.
- Deep nasal breathing. Slowly inhale to fill your lungs with healing oxygen, then slowly exhale through your mouth to release all the carbon dioxide. Repeat until you drift off to sleep.
- Meditation and prayer.

How was your sleep rating on your **Life Balance Foundation** tool? If it is low, I hope this sleep guidance helps you take action to improve the best healing time in your life.

Another way to improve your energy, health, and happiness is to be mindful throughout your day.

CHAPTER 14

Mindfulness

*Open your heart and mind to being in the moment,
a gift of inner peace.*

The journey from worldly pulls to mindfulness has created a wonderful and calming presence in my life. My life is no longer about my selfish pleasures. It's about being centered on the divine purpose of my life, an unselfish presence that took time to achieve. It feels so good to wake up with a smile and say: "Good morning! How can I serve you today, God?"

During my wellness journey, when I finally accepted that my unconscious choices caused me harm, this calmed my fears and hope began to shine its light on me. This hope brought me the courage, determination, and strength to walk the Metanoia path to healing. It was then I began living in the present moment.

Why is it that when we get stuck in our past, depression creeps in and when we constantly focus on the future, fear and anxiety flood our being? Living in the moment, where you are right now, is one of the best places to focus your mind, time, and energy. It's perfectly OK to reflect and plan but to get stuck in the past, or in the future, can rob you of peace, joy, and gratefulness.

To enter into mindfulness, bring your mind and heart to the present moment. Be slow to speak and quick to listen to your internal messages as the worldly pulls try to block peace from your being. Look around you and see all the beautiful gifts God has created for you, especially nature and the kindness, love, and joy of others.

A simple method to being in the moment is to open your left hand that represents the past, then open your right hand that represents the future, and bring them together in a prayer position to represent the present moment. Close your eyes, slowly breathe in healing oxygen to fill your lungs. Slowly exhale, twice as long as you inhaled, and release any built-up emotional debris and all the carbon dioxide in your lungs. As you continue this breathing pattern, slow down your breathing pace even more and connect your heartbeat with your

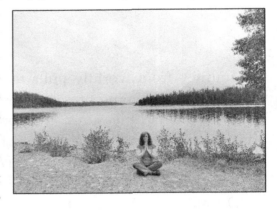

breathing. You will soon feel a calmness in your body, mind, and spirit. You are now in a peaceful and relaxed state. Any built-up barriers will dissolve, your heart rate will reduce, and you can access your highest consciousness with more ease. Practicing this method regularly will help you balance and come back to your true self, especially when you are having a difficult time making a decision due to stress and imbalanced emotions.

MINDFULNESS TO LOSE WEIGHT

Remember it takes 20 minutes for your brain to receive the message that your stomach is full. The slower you consume all food and drinks, the easier you will sense your stomach's fullness. This will help you eat less. If you are a fast and unconscious eater, mindfulness and daily practice will help you create a positive habit of enjoying food at a much slower pace. Doing this may help prevent a future diagnosis of metabolic syndrome, the disease level I reached before my wellness journey.[1] To reverse this disease, I had to acknowledge my bad habit of speed eating while driving from one client's location to another during my medical profession. To do this, I began planning my meals at park picnic tables and restaurants to help me relax, look at the food I was consuming, and slowly enjoy the meal. Another bad habit I had to break was eating while working on the computer. Being unfocused during any snack or mealtime creates overeating, more calorie intake, and weight gain. Here are some more tips that helped me change my negative eating habits into positive ones:

- Focus on your food. Remove yourself from the TV, phone, and computer to enjoy your snack or meal.
- Savor your food. Place a small amount of food on your fork or spoon for each bite and then place the utensil down. When you have finished chewing and swallowing your food, pick up your utensil for another bite. Repeat the process until you are finished eating.
- Pace yourself by taking 10-20 chews before you swallow.

- It's OK to drink water between your bites to help prevent scarfing down your food.
- Eat in moderation. The less you place on your plate, the more you will enjoy what you have to eat. Small portion sizes will help you gauge the amount of food for each meal.
- Eating small frequent and nutritious snacks between meals will curb those extreme hunger pains and reduce speed eating. Consistent eating will also increase your metabolism.

Forming a new habit requires your mind and heart to open up to a new way of life. Replacing a negative habit with a positive habit will always improve your life. The most important thing to remember is to focus on what you want and what you don't want in your life. To help you achieve what you want, adapt the basic components of mindfulness by slowing down, disconnecting from worldly pulls, increasing self-love, surrounding yourself with positive environments and people, and practicing your truth.

CHAPTER 15

Busting Food Addictions

I am not what I have done, I am what I have overcome.

Mr. Carl and Ms. Shoal, former rehab patients, immediately came to my mind when I learned about controversial ingredients. Controversial ingredients are reported to cause neurological diseases, cancer, Multiple Sclerosis, Alzheimer's, headaches, dizziness, diabetes, mood changes, and many other body discomforts and diseases.

Mr. Carl was stiff from his head down to his toes except for the constant tremors that came with his Parkinson's disease, a difficult and incurable neurological disorder. Because he had lost complete body control, he came for medication adjustments and therapy to the nursing home rehab where I worked. He could not feed himself or walk. Each day, little by little, his movements slowly returned as his new medications and therapies were reviving his life. The day he finally fed himself and walked with a walker was a day of celebration! His journey with Parkinson's did not diminish his joy, even though he faced a lifetime of medications and possible setbacks. The light I always saw in Mr. Carl was his strong hope and faith. In time, Mr. Carl did go home, and as he walked out of the facility waving goodbye to his therapy and nursing team, we all waved goodbye with grateful hearts to witness his healing.

Ms. Shoal could barely hold her head up as she tried to brush her hair. Her loose handgrip and wavering arm made it difficult to stroke her hair with the brush. She had been diagnosed with breast cancer and came to the rehab facility because her body became spastic and uncontrollable after receiving multiple radiation treatments. I was told that she had received too much radiation. My heart broke as I watched her glance into the mirror trying to recognize her reflection. She was in an emotional deep fog and tears began to roll down Ms. Shoal's face as she described her life before the breast cancer diagnosis and radiation treatments. We were the same age, 40 years old, and she previously had had an active and full life. My heart's deep compassion continues for her as I reflect on our last goodbye smile to one another. There, but for the grace of God, go I.

What caused these patients' health situations? Was it their genetic disposition, lifestyle, environmental exposures, food choices, or was it fate?

When fear erupted in my soul after learning aspartame was in the Diet Dr. Pepper and sugar-free chewing gum I consumed each day, I had to take action to protect my health. Releasing all controversial ingredients from my body was one of the first action steps to busting my food and drink addictions. To my surprise, quitting sugar-free chewing gum was an easy cold turkey event. Weaning from Diet Dr. Pepper took a bit longer. Because I knew that water is the best fluid for the body, I created a diet soda detox process using a mixture of water and Diet Dr.

Pepper. On day one, I filled my glass with 2/3 soda drink and 1/3 water. The soda drink flavor was still sweet and flavorful, so I drank it that way for a couple of days.

Step #2 in my detox process included a glass filled with 50/50% water/diet soda combination. Enjoying the diet soda flavor mixed with water helped ease my addiction cravings while offering my body chemistry a chance to rebalance and strengthen. This solution was good for several days until step #3 detox process became a 25% soda and 75% water combination. Within two weeks Diet Dr. Pepper was completely weaned from my life! From that experience came a nutritious habit of adding fresh-squeezed juice or slices of my favorite fresh fruit, vegetables, or some flavorful spices to a glass of water. You too can wean yourself from soda drinks if your energy, health, and happiness are something you truly value and do not want to compromise.

After busting these two major addictions, the next plan of action was to empower my body with moderate amounts of nutritious whole clean foods: fresh fruits, vegetables, whole grains, nuts, seeds, healthy fats, and diverse protein foods. Simple and easy home cooking became a daily habit and continues to be to this day. I enjoy new food recipe adventures and sharing them with family, friends, and clients.

Instead of reaching for my favorite Snickers bar, I now reach for a couple of nuts and fruit. Some days, I'll even make a peanut butter, banana, and seed creation to nix a sweet craving. The Starbucks frozen coffee drink I used to crave is now replaced with a frozen banana cocoa milkshake or a frozen fruit treat. These healthy substitutes offer delicious flavors and a nutritional energy boost!

As you read in Chapter 10, "Clean Is Supreme," controversial products can deplete vital micronutrients and hijack your body's energy and wellbeing. When these products are regularly overconsumed, in time, disease may enter the body. If you have children or grandchildren, please honor their health and offer them clean whole foods and water. You are the example they will follow with their daily habits, drink, and food choices.

Below are additional wellness resources to empower your daily choices and to help you gain more prevention and reversal tips.

- Dr. Ornish, cardiovascular disease reversal:
  https://www.ornish.com/proven-program/nutrition/
- Dr. Furhman, diabetes reversal:
  https://www.drfuhrman.com/
- D. Daniel Amen, improve brain and body function:
  danielamenmd.com
- American Heart Association: **www.heart.org**
- American Diabetes Association: **www.diabetes.org**
- American Cancer Organization: **www.cancer.org**

CHAPTER 16

Get SMART, Get Ready, Go!

*Goals are dreams we convert into plans and
take action to fulfill — Zig Ziglar*

There on the bathroom mirror hung a bright yellow sticky note with my handwritten goals. I stared deeply at this small piece of paper, stimulating and focusing my brain every single day and night. Every time I went to the bathroom sink to wash my hands, brush my hair, wash my face, and brush my teeth, the sticky note reminded me of what I wanted to accomplish in my life. Once the goals were accomplished, I replaced that sticky note with a fresh one and new written goals. I'm not sure where I learned this simple and successful method, but it's worked for me since 1994 when I became a single mother.

To create change in your life, you must know what you value, what you want, and what you don't want in your life. Once you discover that, write down your top three life goals. If you want to try the sticky note method, briefly write them in order of importance and stick your note where you will see it first thing in the morning, multiple times a day, and right before you go to bed. The bathroom mirror was the best place for me to place my sticky notes because my brain could focus 100% on my written goals.

Once your goals are written down, being smart will help you get what you want a lot faster. Take a look at these S.M.A.R.T. tips to help you get there.

S – SPECIFIC goals will help you manage your time. On a piece of paper, or in your journal, write down why you want to achieve your goals, when the best time is to start your action, and where you need to be to accomplish your goals. Who do you need to help you get there? The more specific you are, the less time you will waste.

M – Make your goals MEASURABLE by writing them down and what necessary steps you need to take. Checking off your accomplishments as you journey toward your goals is a wonderful feeling!

A – What is your heart's desire and future life vision? Do your goals match them? If your goals support them, they are more ATTAINABLE.

R – Are your goals REALISTIC? Some people may be too strict with their goals at the beginning of a wellness journey. When our mind and heart opens to learning new ways of doing things, it allows us to make daily adjustments and become more realistic with our goals.

T – Having a deadline to reach your goals will help fuel your determination and perseverance to achieve TIMELY goals. However, if circumstances out of your control prevent you from reaching your deadline, it's OK to reset it. If this happens, you are not a failure; you are being wise to accommodate time to handle other life callings. You can make readjustments as needed to accomplish what you want in life.

Having a trusted accountability partner will be a powerful support as you travel your wellness journey, especially if life derails your best intentions with unexpected situations. If this happens, contact your accountability partner and get the support you need. The world is constantly changing around us. Being able to adapt to changes will help you maintain balance on your wellness journey. Unexpected life circumstances can happen to any of us, any time, and without notice.

TIPS TO PONDER

- Examples of life's unexpected happenings include: the Covid pandemic, the birth of a new family member, a marriage, or even a sudden loss of something or someone you value (i.e., death of a family member or a friend, divorce, sickness, losing a job, or an accident).
- Worldly temptations are everywhere! The more balanced you are in life, the less worldly temptations will divert

you. If you have a difficult time getting back on track, go back and review your goals. You may want to update your **Life Balance Foundation** tool in Chapter 2 and review your **Time Wheel** in Chapter 5 to see if you have any unnoticed imbalances.

- Mindless time zappers will rob your precious time. Social media, TV, and the internet are some big culprits in this area. If you want these connections in your life, offer yourself a controlled amount of time to enjoy them so they won't divert your time and energy from achieving your goals.

Reflect on what truly warms your heart and fills your soul. All the positive things that feed your soul and generate a warm glow throughout your entire being will provide you with more energy, health, and happiness. This will also radiate positive energy to others.

As you awaken, the tone of your day is being set. A morning ritual that offers your body, mind, and spirit a pleasant and calm beginning provides more peace in your day. Some positive ideas include waking up in time to:

- Reflect on what you are grateful for.
- Express your feelings and write them in a journal.
- Spend a few minutes doing centering prayer, meditation, deep breathing along with light yoga, Qigong, or simple stretches.
- Sip a warm cup of water with fresh-squeezed lemon or minced ginger root, or green tea.
- Create and enjoy a nutritious breakfast.

Making yourself a priority is essential for self-love and being available to others. Each day, living from the center of love makes it easier to live your truth and your values and to honor and respect yourself. When you do this, what you want in life will find its way to you. Be patient and live each moment to the fullest.

A beautiful thing about life is your ability to change, grow, and heal. You are not defined by your past or your mistakes.

My wish for you is to have what you want in life. May you be blessed with joyful wellness!

Simple Nutritious Recipes

You can't go back and change the beginning, but you can start where you are and change the ending. — C.S. Lewis

My hope for you is that you gain knowledge to discover new food choices to replace the unhealthy ones that fuel unconscious cravings and addiction.

We all have a unique set of taste buds and biochemistry, so no one food will satisfy everybody. You are the only one who can decide what works for your taste buds and your body. Adapting to new foods may take several attempts, although when clean whole foods are introduced into your body, they will improve your body's chemistry, help decrease cravings, lift your moods, and empower you with better energy and health benefits.

Choosing nutritious foods when you are away from home is vital for a successful wellness journey. When walking on the Metanoia path, you may slip into old habits. Try not to beat yourself up. Get back up, dust yourself off, forgive yourself, and keep moving forward with your clean nutritious ways. Focus on your goals and what you want in life.

Making time for new food adventures can be fun, exciting, simple, and easy. The more snacks and meals prepared at home, the easier this pattern will turn into positive habits and help you create a bounty of go-to-recipes. Family and friends will enjoy sharing the results with you as you try out new recipes created in your kitchen. Once they give the recipe a thumbs up, place it in a recipe binder and share it with others.

The recipes shared in this chapter were a major part of my wellness journey and are used to this day. These recipes, plus more, are kept in a large spiral binder in my kitchen cabinet. Each recipe is documented with a grade, the date it was created, and any changes or additions from the original recipe.

Remember, the past is behind you. It's time to live in the moment as you walk toward your new life. Happy yummy adventures to you and yours!

CLEAN PRODUCE BEFORE YOU BITE

Organic does not mean it's clean of bugs, dirt, and bacteria. Fresh produce is touched by many unclean hands and sits on grocery counters that may add germs and bacteria. Cleaning all fresh vegetables and fruit before eating, cooking, or freezing is a healthy practice and worth the time for your best health. A water-vinegar soak solution is a way I clean all purchased fresh produce before it's eaten raw, cooked, or before freezing. For example, I place all the leaves from a head of romaine lettuce in a large container, or clean sink, with 12 cups of water and 1/2 cup of white vinegar. Then, I stir the mixture for 30 seconds and let them

CHAPTER 17

soak for 5 – 10 minutes. Next, I rinse each leaf individually under the faucet and place it on a towel to dry, or pour out the dirty water and fill the container again with fresh water over the romaine lettuce leaves. I swish the leaves around again to remove any remaining bugs, dirt, or debris. Next, I dump out the dirty water and do a final and third repeat of filling the container with fresh water and the romaine leaves. I do a final swish with the leaves, remove the water, and place the leaves in a colander to drip dry, or on a towel, then pat dry.

HOME COOKING METHODS

Adventuring with different cooking methods has helped me increase more nutritious whole foods into my daily meals and snacks. An investment of time was required to discover the taste and texture of new foods that eventually replaced the destructive choices I used to eat. Giving up social media, TV, and mindless activities was not a problem to begin home cooking. I wanted more than anything in life to have good health and for my life to be filled with joy, peace, and happiness.

The main cooking methods I use to this day include steamed, stir-fried, baked, roasted, blanched, and quick microwaving. Recipes can be created, shared by family and friends, found in magazines, newspapers, the internet, and cookbooks. To get a break from daily cooking, I prepare large amounts of a recipe and freeze leftovers for future meals and snacks. For example, when I bake a whole chicken, the breast and other parts can be used in a recipe or frozen for later creations, casseroles, chili, and soup. After the chicken meat is eaten, I place all the bones are in a large gallon freezer bag and freeze them to make broth at a later date.

SWEET NUTRITIOUS SUBSTITUTES AND RECIPES!

Choosing nutritious sugar replacements was easy, fun to create, and rewarding! If you are keeping an eye on your calorie intake, weight, and glucose levels, know that dried fruit's nutrient, calorie, and fructose levels are more condensed than fresh fruit. Researching fructose differences will help you decide your best serving size. Below are a few of my favorite nutritious sweet choices. These recipes helped me walk the Metanoia path to healing. Keep in mind the moderate serving and portion sizes for each meal and snack.

- Organic fresh and frozen whole fruit of all kinds.
- Organic frozen grapes. Red and dark-colored grapes offer the most resveratrol and phytonutrients.
- Fresh organic Gala apple sprinkled with cinnamon. Add organic peanut butter to the side for a yummy protein dip.
- Occasional Majool dates and raisins, in moderation.

INFUSED WATER

Infused water is a nutritious replacement for sodas, other processed drinks, and an easy way to increase your water intake.

Place one or more fresh pieces of whole fruit, vegetable, or herb into a pitcher or a glass of water. Place in the refrigerator for one hour to absorb the plant flavors. When you finish drinking, the remaining fruit, veggie, and herb can be a great snack!

The following are some choices for infused water: Apples, oranges, strawberries, cucumbers, lemons, limes, grapefruit, watermelon, kiwi, berries, cherries, fresh mint, basil, ginger, rosemary, and cinnamon sticks.

SUGAR DE-CRAVER MILKSHAKE

This delicious creation was made using a $25 Oster blender. It satisfied my uncontrollable sweet cravings and helped me bust sugar addiction.

½ cup frozen organic blueberries
4 frozen organic strawberries
1/2 quartered frozen banana
1 cup unsweetened almond milk or organic pasture-raised milk

Add all ingredients to the blender and blend at the slowest speed. Stop blender and stir when needed. Enjoy this sweet treat using a spoon, straw, or simply drinking from a tall glass.

WELLNESS SMOOTHIE

This smoothie provides lots of micronutrients for an energy boost!

One inch slice of fresh or frozen ginger
1-2 organic cooked frozen Lucinato kale leaves
1/4 cup frozen organic or wild blueberries
2-3 organic frozen strawberries
1/2 quartered frozen banana
2 TBSP fresh or frozen pineapple
1/2 cup organic Greek yogurt
1 cup water (or 1/2 cup organic pasture-raised milk + 1/2 cup water)

Add all ingredients to a blender and blend until liquidized. Adjust the recipe to your taste buds.

CHOCOLATE BANANA MILKSHAKE

1 quartered frozen banana
1/4 - 1/2 cup organic pasture-raised milk or milk of choice
1 tsp. cocoa powder

Mix in a blender. (Adjust blender speed and milk for desired consistency.)

WATERMELON POPSICLES

Blend 4 cups of fresh seedless watermelon in a blender and pour into BPA-free popsicle containers. Freeze until firm. (Optional: Add fresh chopped mint for added nutrition and flavor.)

SWEET CRUNCHY SEED CREATION

Perfect for a single serving snack. Seeds offer your body protein, healthy fats, and many micronutrients.

In a small bowl mix the following ingredients with a fork and eat the treat from the bowl:

1/2 ripe banana (mash and stir with a fork)
1/2 TBSP organic peanut butter
1/2 tsp ground flaxseed (optional)
1 tsp sunflower seeds (optional)
1 tsp pepita seeds

FROZEN BANANA TREAT

Each week I purchase a bunch of ripe bananas, slice them into small quarter bite-size pieces, then place them in a container in the freezer for smoothies and this treat. This is a yummy ice cream substitute.

1 quartered frozen banana
5 broken or chopped pecans
1 teaspoon honey
Cinnamon (optional)

Place frozen quartered banana in decorative glass for ambiance (I use a blue martini glass). Top with pecans and sprinkle with cinnamon. Pour honey over the top of all ingredients.

CRUNCHY FRUIT YOGURT TREAT

This satisfies a sweet tooth and fills your body with powerhouse nutrients.

1/2 cup frozen organic cherries
1/2 cup frozen organic blueberries
1/2 cup organic Greek Yogurt
1 TBSP pepita seeds

Place cherries and blueberries in a bowl. Allow to semi-thaw for 15 minutes or place in microwave for 30 seconds. Top fruit with organic Greek yogurt. Sprinkle yogurt with pepita seeds. (Optional: Add 5 chopped almonds for additional protein.)

SAUTÉED APPLES

This tasty side dish or dessert is a family favorite passed down from my Appalachian heritage. It's a joy to share this during family and friendship meals.

Slice and seed 5-7 organic apples (Gala or Granny Smith). Keep the skin on the apples as it is rich in fiber, micronutrients, and antioxidants.

Heat 10" skillet on medium-high. Add 1 – 2 TBSP organic pasture-raised butter. Add sliced apples, stir and sauté until apples soften, approximately 5-8 minutes. Lower heat as needed. Add a little water if apples stick to the pan while sautéing. Sprinkle lightly with cinnamon.

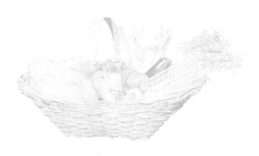

QUICK POPCORN SNACKS

An airless popcorn popper creates a quick nutritious snack with minimal clean-up. Popcorn, a whole grain, offers your body nutritious fiber and many micronutrients. Enjoy your popcorn plain or adventure with some flavors. For a five-cup serving, add 2 TBSP organic popcorn to an airless popcorn popper with a large bowl placed underneath the spout. Pop until done. Yum!

For all the flavors below, mix the ingredients in a small cup and stir until blended. Add the ingredients to five cups of popped popcorn in a large bowl. Stir the mixture with a large spoon until popcorn is coated.

SWEET FLAVOR:
1 TBSP organic pasture-raised melted butter or olive oil
1 tsp honey
1/8 tsp cinnamon (optional - adjust to your palette)

CHEESY FLAVOR
1 TBSP olive oil
1 tsp Nutritional Yeast (adjust to your palette)

LEMON PEPPER FLAVOR
Mix 1 TBSP olive oil
1/2 - 1 tsp lemon pepper seasoning (adjust to your palette)

SEED TOAST

Very easy to make! Start with any bread you choose, then follow the ingredient order when creating this nutritious protein combination.

1 slice of toasted bread of your choice
1 TBSP organic peanut butter or almond butter, spread on toast, then add:

> 1 tsp honey (spread evenly over peanut butter)
> Sprinkle lightly with cinnamon and top with seeds.
> 1/2 tsp ground flaxseed
> 1/2 tsp sesame seeds (optional)
> 1/2 tsp sunflower seeds
> 2 tsp pepita seeds

Pat all seeds down with a knife into the peanut butter honey mixture. Slice in half. Enjoy!

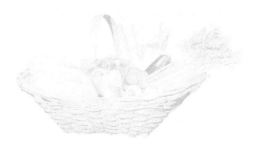

MEXICAN BOILED EGGS

Easy and quick protein breakfast! Two eggs per person. Enjoy with sliced avocado and organic sweet red pepper.

Place organic pasture-raised eggs in a pot and cover with water. Heat on high until boiling. Lower heat for a slow 10-minute boil. Remove from heat. Allow eggs to cool or place in cold water. When cooled, and ready to eat, peel eggs and cut into quarters. If you are watching your cholesterol levels, dispose one of the yokes.

Top eggs with:
1-2 TBSP organic salsa of choice
1 TBSP Fresh chopped cilantro

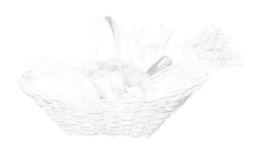

OATMEAL

Oatmeal is a filling breakfast or pre-bedtime choice. It can be cooked on the stove or in a microwave. Choose your favorite nuts, seeds, fruit, and liquid to satisfy your taste buds and nutrition needs. My favorite combination includes organic whole rolled oats, raisins, pepita seeds, and organic pasture-raised milk.

TO COOK ON STOVE TOP:
Add 1 cup water to a small pot. Turn the heat on high. Once the water begins to boil, reduce the heat to low and add 1/2 cup organic whole rolled oats. Stir for approximately 5 minutes to prevent oats from sticking to the bottom of the pan. Turn off the heat and remove the pan. Place a lid on the pan for a minute. Scoop desired oatmeal into a bowl adding your choice of fruit, nuts, seeds, and liquid to create your tastiest oatmeal.

TO COOK IN THE MICROWAVE:
For one serving, place one handful of whole organic rolled oats into a bowl, cover with water, then stir. Place bowl in the microwave for 45 – 60 seconds. Add your favorite fruit, nuts, seeds, and liquid.

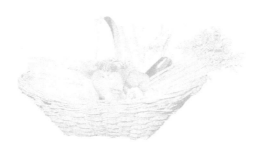

Pam Frazier, INHC

HOMEMADE HUMMUS

Nutritious and delicious protein dip enjoyed with sliced carrots, celery, cucumber, peppers, radishes, or organic corn chips.

1 ½ cups cooked or canned whole garbanzo beans
3 cloves garlic, minced
2 TBSP Tahini
1 TBSP olive oil
1 tsp paprika
Juice ½ lemon
½ tsp cumin
½ tsp sea salt
¼ - ½ cup water (add as you blend other ingredients)

Add all ingredients to a blender and slowly blend while adding water for desired consistency. Enjoy!

ROASTED SWEET POTATOES
A delicious and nutritious favorite!

6-8 Sweet potatoes
coconut oil
cinnamon
chopped pecans (optional)

Pre-heat oven to 350 degrees. Lightly hand rub all potatoes with a light coating of coconut oil. Slice potatoes in half, lengthwise. Place open sliced potatoes face down in a 3-quart casserole dish. Bake 35 minutes. Serve with a light sprinkling of cinnamon and pecans on top of each sweet potato serving.

OVEN-ROASTED POTATOES

Delicious and nutritious substitute for French fries.

Mix all ingredients in a large bowl:
2 TBSP olive oil
1 TBSP minced garlic
1/2 tsp dried basil
1/2 tsp dill weed
1/2 tsp dried thyme
1/2 tsp dried oregano
1 tsp sea salt

Add:
6 large organic potatoes cut in 2-inch quartered pieces (red, russet, or mix with sweet potatoes) and hand toss or stir until potatoes are evenly coated.

Directions:
1. Preheat oven to 475 degrees
2. Place coated potatoes in a single layer on a baking sheet.
3. Bake @ 475 for 25 - 30 minutes – occasionally turn to brown all sides.

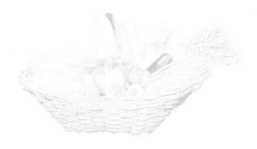

EASY HOMEMADE VEGGIE PIZZA

Family and friends enjoy making their pizza when we gather in the kitchen. This pizza has very low sodium and sugar content compared to most pizza restaurants. It's quick, nutritious, and fun!

Use pita bread, artisan flatbread, or cauliflower pizza crust for the base.

1-2 TBSP organic pizza sauce per piece* (spread over bread)
1/8 tsp basil and oregano (sprinkle over sauce)
1/8 tsp garlic powder (sprinkle over sauce)
1/4 - 1/3 cup shredded mozzarella cheese

Layer your choice of veggies over the prepared bread and cheese.

1/4 cup sliced fresh mushrooms
1-2 TBSP chopped onions
2 TBSP chopped green or red pepper
4-6 fresh basil leaves

Preheat oven to 425 degrees.
Place pizza in the oven for 10 minutes.
Slice with a pizza cutter. Enjoy!

* Freeze any remaining pizza sauce in ice cube trays for future pizza makings.

GRILLED CHEESE WITH TOMATO & ONION

Griddler by Cuisinart is a simple tool I use to make this grilled sandwich. Family and friends enjoy them and always want more!

Set the Griddler on 400 degrees plus the Grilled Panini and Sear settings.

Per sandwich use:
2 slices of your choice of bread
1 organic slice of cheese
organic mayonnaise
organic tomato, sliced
1 slice of purple onion, cut up

Spread bread slices with a light coating of mayonnaise. On one slice of bread add cheese, purple onion, and 1-3 tomato slices. Cover with the other slice of bread and place the sandwich on the Griddler when the sear light has turned green. Cook until cheese melts and the bread is lightly browned.

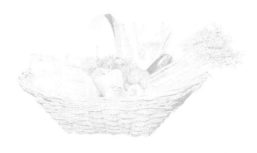

CHICKEN FAJITAS

A nutritious meal pleaser for 4 people!

Ingredients:
1 pound of boneless organic chicken breast (skinless and thinly sliced)
1 large organic red pepper (seeded and thinly sliced)
1 large organic yellow or orange pepper (seeded and thinly sliced)
1 purple onion (halved and thinly sliced)

Marinade ingredients:
3 TBSP fresh squeezed lime juice
1 TBSP olive oil
2 TBSP finely chopped fresh cilantro
1 TBSP minced garlic
1 1/2 TBSP organic low sodium soy sauce
1 tsp honey
1/2 tsp cumin
1/2 tsp chili powder

Place marinade ingredients in a medium bowl and stir. Add chicken to marinade and stir, thoroughly coating the chicken. Let stand in the refrigerator for at least 15 minutes. Add peppers and onion to the chicken marinade and stir well.

Place mixture on a large rimmed baking sheet. Bake at 400 degrees for 25-30 minutes, or until chicken is cooked through. Place 1/2 cup of mixture in a flour tortilla and fold over for a delicious fajita!

CHICKEN BROTH

Homemade chicken broth is easy and economical. The longer you cook the broth, the more nutrients will flow into your broth. Place bones of one chicken into a 7-quart crockpot. Add the following ingredients:

1 chopped white onion
3 chopped large carrots
3 chopped celery sticks with leaves
3 garlic cloves
2 tsp black peppercorns
2 bay leaves

Place all ingredients in the crockpot, fill it with water. Cover and cook on high for 8 hours.

Turn heat to low and cook an additional 16 hours. Allow broth to cool in the crockpot container then place the container in the refrigerator for several hours. When the broth has chilled, discard the bones and vegetables. Strain broth into a large bowl using a sifter covered with cheesecloth. This will collect any leftover fat and thick substance. Rinse out cheesecloth as needed and continue to drain the rest of the broth into the bowl or an additional bowl. Broth can be stored in a refrigerator for a couple of days or placed in a freezer container for later use. Pint and quart size containers work well.

HEALING SOUP

This is the best soup to enjoy when you feel a cold, cough or low energy creeping into your day. Made with love and immunity-boosting ingredients.

Ingredients:
6 cups chicken broth
One 2-inch fresh ginger, finely chopped
4 sliced green onions, 1-inch pieces
1-2 minced garlic cloves
3/4 cup thinly sliced mushrooms

Place vegetables in a pot with 1/2 cup of broth. Simmer until ingredients are softened. Add the remaining broth and bring to a boil. Reduce heat and simmer for 30 minutes.

SALMON WITH BLACK BEANS

High protein fiber meal! The perfect mix with a green salad. For each serving, place a 4 oz piece of Wild Alaskan salmon on a wire rack placed over a parchment paper-covered pan. Cook at 450 degrees 10 – 15 minutes. Peel the skin off the cooked salmon using a fork and place the salmon on a plate. Top with 1/4 to 1/2 cup of warm black beans. Top with 1/4 cup of your favorite salsa and sprinkle with fresh cilantro.

YUMMY TUNA SALAD

Packed with protein, probiotics, vitamin C, and potassium!

1 can wild-caught tuna, drained
1 diced celery stalk
1/4 cup onion of choice (white, purple, or green onions)
2-3 finely chopped small dill pickles
1 TBSP fresh squeezed lemon juice
1 clove minced garlic
1/4 – 1/3 cup organic mayonnaise

Stir and mix all ingredients. Enjoy as a burrito, sandwich, or with a side salad.

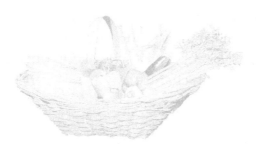

In Gratitude

All the people I have met in my life have gifted me a special seed. These seeds have bloomed into a smile, heart connection, friendship, love, lesson, wisdom, an avenue to self-awareness, growth, and reunion with God. I thank you all!

Grounded in faith, my desire to heal required an open-minded physician and medical team who agreed to support my wellness journey. In perfect time, our paths crossed during a professional breakfast meeting. From that day forward, my heart is full of gratefulness to Faith Johnson, CRNP, and Cindy McAdams, DO. With the support of this awesome medical team, I walked away from three physicians who offered me no hope of self-healing, only a life of medications and a recommendation for thyroid removal.

Ten years before, my days were filled with unconscious habits and misguided choices. I was led astray by the darkness of worldly pulls. All of this contributed to a flood of stress, poor nutrition, and an imbalanced life. My self-awareness was blinded, and my relationship with my divine rock, God, was minimal. These factors affected my health, stripped my peace, and wasted precious time.

In addition to a supportive medical team, my wellness journey also included three enlightening books that made their unique path to me within months of each other.

The first book, *Anatomy of the Spirit*, by Carolyn Myss, was gifted to me by my dear friend, Dr. David Lehner. Carolyn Myss's words and wisdom helped me get in touch with my inner self and God. This began my self-love journey. I am forever grateful to you my dear friend, Dave, and Carolyn Myss.

The second book, *Younger Next Year for Women*, by Chris Crowley and Dr. Henry S. Lodge, flashed its hot pink cover at me a couple of times as I looked around the airport gift shop in Ontario, California. This book helped me renew my vitality oath and create a vision for successful aging.

The third book, *The Sugar Smart Diet*, written by Anne Alexander, was suggested to me in a marketing letter from Prevention magazine. This education opened my mind to busting my sugar addiction. Thank you all at Prevention magazine for your wonderful wellness guidance.

Thank you to Joshua Rosenthal, founder of the Institute of Integrative Nutrition, my 2015 alma mater. Your inspiring education enlightened my mind, my heart, my health, and my life!

Thank you to my daughter Melissa Goldman; Nell Richardson; Barb Mandeville; Lynda Walker; Tim and Miriam Ezell; Angela Peratta; Alberta Cooley; my brother Larry, Jr; Cindy Martin; graphic artist, Angi at C&A Printing; my editor, Sammie Barstow; and designer, Ellen Maze Sallas for all your support and guidance during this long book project. Thank you Canva for the ability to use your free platform and images.

The mystical power of God receives 100% credit for all these connections and blessings of guidance, education, and inspiration. I am eternally grateful for all who shared from their hearts and unknowingly took part in my wellness journey.

Within four months after hearing Pastor Joy Nellissery's question, "How are you treating your holy temple?" I was able to discontinue the blood pressure and thyroid medications and the thyroid surgery was never scheduled. To this day, my thyroid is intact, and my focus radiates a life of joyful wellness.

When I heard God's spiritual message, "Pam, do not be afraid," I knew it was time to inspire, educate, and guide others to a life of joyful wellness. God wants you to love your holy temple as He loves you.

With a grateful and humble heart, it's been an honor to witness people transform their lives as they began making wiser choices when they discovered their Metanoia path. Many have reversed disease in their own life. As their wellness journey continues, they become inspiring mentors for all in their world who witness their transformation. Without knowing it, they are spreading many seeds to help create more blooms in our world.

I hope you are gifted from the seeds in this book and plant them within your garden of life.

Much love,
Pam Frazier

CHAPTER 1: AWAKENED

"The flower doesn't dream of the bee. It blossoms and the bee comes" quote "by Mark Nepo, from The Book of Awakening © 2020, 2011, 2000.May 19 passage, page 165

1. https://www.cdc.gov/obesity/index.html US obesity 10.10.20
2. https://www.cdc.gov/heartdisease/facts.htm 10.10.20
3. https://www.cdc.gov/chronicdisease/about/prevent/index. htm 10.10.20
4. https://healthcare.utah.edu/the-scope/shows.php?shows=0_smfdnnqq Dr. Kirtly Parker Jones 8.4.20
5. https://pubmed.ncbi.nlm.nih.gov/17698405/ Clore GL, Huntsinger JR. How emotions inform judgment and regulate thought. Trends Cogn Sci. 2007 Sep;11(9):393-9. doi: 10.1016/j.tics.2007.08.005. Epub 2007 Aug 16. PMID: 17698405; PMCID: PMC2483304.
6. "American Geriatrics Society Updated Beers Criteria®." www.GeriatricsCareOnline.org, American Geriatrics Society. January 31, 2019. geriatricscareonline.org/toc/american-geriatrics-society-updated-beers-criteria/CL001 9.30.20

CHAPTER 2: AWARENESS – THE FOUNDATION OF CHANGE

1. No Man is an Island, by Thomas Merton, 1955. Permission granted by the Merton Legacy Trust. 7.16.20
2. https://www.ninds.nih.gov/Disorders/Patient-Caregiver-Education/Understanding-Sleep 7.20.20

3. https://www.ncbi.nlm.nih.gov/pmc/articles/PMC5768235/ 7.20.20

4. https://pubmed.ncbi.nlm.nih.gov/24214244/ Park DC, Lodi-Smith J, Drew L, Haber S, Hebrank A, Bischof GN, Aamodt W. The impact of sustained engagement on cognitive function in older adults: the Synapse Project. Psychol Sci. 2014 Jan;25(1):103-12. doi: 10.1177/0956797613499592. Epub 2013 Nov 8. PMID: 24214244; PMCID: PMC4154531.

CHAPTER 4: UNDERSTAND EPIGENETICS

1. https://www.genome.gov/genetics-glossary/Epigenetics , Laura Elnitski, Ph.D. at The National Human Genome Research Institute 8.11.20

2. https://pubmed.ncbi.nlm.nih.gov/30202288/ Buettner D, Skemp S. Blue Zones: Lessons From the World's Longest Lived. Am J Lifestyle Med. 2016;10(5):318-321. Published 2016 Jul 7. doi:10.1177/1559827616637066 8.12.20

3. https://pubmed.ncbi.nlm.nih.gov/27053941/ Passarino G, De Rango F, Montesanto A. Human longevity: Genetics or Lifestyle? It takes two to tango. Immun Ageing. 2016;13:12. Published 2016 Apr 5. doi:10.1186/s12979-016-0066-z 8.21.20

CHAPTER 5: BEGINNING A WELLNESS JOURNEY

1. Harvey Mackay author of the #1 New York Times bestseller, "Swim With the Sharks Without Being Eaten Alive" Permission granted 7.15.20

CHAPTER 6: YOU ARE A MIRACLE

1. https://www.usgs.gov/special-topic/water-science-school/science/water-you-water-and-human-body?qt-science_center_objects=0#qt-science_center_objects 7.8.21
2. https://www.fda.gov/consumers/consumer-updates/fda-101-dietary-supplements 6.1.21
3. https://training.seer.cancer.gov/anatomy/body/ 6.4.21
4. https://www.cdc.gov/nceh/publications/books/housing/cha05.htm dust mites 7.21.21
5. https://www.hhs.gov/programs/topic-sites/sexually-transmitted-infections/resources/index.html 6.7.21
6. https://www.niaid.nih.gov/research/immune-system-overview 6.7.21

The Human Body Atlas, by Professor Ken Ashwell BMEDSC, MBBS, PHD. 2016 Chartwell Books

CHAPTER 7: STRESS CAN DO WHAT TO ME??!!

1. https://pubmed.ncbi.nlm.nih.gov/23403892/ Nerurkar A, Bitton A, Davis RB, Phillips RS, Yeh G. When physicians counsel about stress: results of a national study. JAMA Intern Med. 2013 Jan 14;173(1):76-7. doi: 10.1001/2013.jamainternmed.480. PMID: 23403892; PMCID: PMC4286362. 6.10.21
2. https://journals.plos.org/plosone/article?id=10.1371/journal.pone.0000698 6.10.21
3. https://www.ncbi.nlm.nih.gov/pmc/articles/PMC3228640/ Mitchell NS, Catenacci VA, Wyatt HR, Hill JO. Obesity: overview of an epidemic. Psychiatr Clin North Am. 2011 Dec;34(4):717-32. doi: 10.1016/j.psc.2011.08.005. PMID: 22098799; PMCID: PMC3228640. 6.10.21
4. https://www.nih.gov/news-events/nih-research-matters/stress-may-awaken-dormant-cancer-cells 1.13.21

5. https://www.cdc.gov/nceh/default.htm National Center For Environmental Health 6.10.21

6. https://www.cdc.gov/populationhealth/well-being/ Emotional Well-Being – Population Health 6.10.21

7. https://pubmed.ncbi.nlm.nih.gov/25898780/ Hemmingsen JG, Møller P, Jantzen K, Jönsson BA, Albin M, Wierzbicka A, Gudmundsson A, Loft S, Rissler J. Controlled exposure to diesel exhaust and traffic noise-- Effects on oxidative stress and activation in mononuclear blood cells. Mutat Res. 2015 May; 775:66-71. doi: 10.1016/j.mrfmmm.2015.03.009. Epub 2015 Mar 28. PMID: 25898780. 6.10.21

8. https://www.cdc.gov/workplacehealthpromotion/index.h tml Work Place Health Promotion 6.10.21

9. https://www.cdc.gov/niosh/docs/99-101/default.html The National Institute for Occupational Safety and Health (NIOSH) 6.10.21

CHAPTER 8: YOUR FOOD CHOICES MATTER

1. https://www.ers.usda.gov/data-products/chart-gallery/gallery/chartdetail/?chartId=58340#:~:text=Potatoe s%20and%20tomatoes%20are%20the,consumption%20aft er%20adjusting%20for%20losses. 7.29.20

2. https://www.fs.fed.us/wildflowers/ethnobotany/medicin al/index.shtml 6.11.21

3. https://www.fs.fed.us/wildflowers/ethnobotany/docume nts/HowPlantsProtectUs.pdf 6.11.21

4. https://www.fs.fed.us/wildflowers/ethnobotany/medicin al/index.shtml 6.11.21

5. https://www.accessdata.fda.gov/scripts/interactivenutriti onfactslabel/assets/InteractiveNFL_TotalCarbohydrate_ March2020.pdf carbohydrates 6.11.21

6. https://wholegrainscouncil.org/what-whole-grain 8.5.20
7. https://www.accessdata.fda.gov/scripts/interactivenutriti onfactslabel/assets/InteractiveNFL_Protein_March2020.p df 6.20.21
8. https://www.nal.usda.gov/fnic/dri-calculator/ 8.20.21
9. https://www.nal.usda.gov/sites/www.nal.usda.gov/files/ protein.pdf 6.20.21
10. https://www.accessdata.fda.gov/scripts/interactivenutriti onfactslabel/assets/InteractiveNFL_TotalFat_March2020. pdf fat 6.20.21
11. https://pubmed.ncbi.nlm.nih.gov/32581851/ Lipids constitute the bulk of the dry mass of the brain and have been associated with healthy function as well as the most common pathological conditions of the brain. 6.28.21
12. https://www.heart.org/en/healthy-living/healthy-eating/eat-smart/fats/dietary-fats 6.20.21
13. https://www.accessdata.fda.gov/scripts/InteractiveNutriti onFactsLabel/vitamins.cfm 6.23.21
14. https://www.niddk.nih.gov/health-information/liver-disease/hemochromatosis 6.25.21
15. https://ods.od.nih.gov/factsheets/VitaminC-HealthProfessional/ 6.25.21
16. https://ods.od.nih.gov/factsheets/VitaminC-HealthProfessional/#h3 mg VC foods 6.25.21
17. https://pubmed.ncbi.nlm.nih.gov/21076725/ Spence JD, Jenkins DJ, Davignon J. Dietary cholesterol and egg yolks: not for patients at risk of vascular disease. Can J Cardiol. 2010 Nov;26(9):e336-9. doi: 10.1016/s0828-282x(10)70456-6. PMID: 21076725; PMCID: PMC2989358. 6.28.21
18. https://pubmed.ncbi.nlm.nih.gov/23666469/ Lorenz EC, Michet CJ, Milliner DS, Lieske JC. Update on oxalate

crystal disease. Curr Rheumatol Rep. 2013 Jul;15(7):340. doi: 10.1007/s11926-013-0340-4. PMID: 23666469; PMCID: PMC3710657. 6.28.21

Macronutrient, vitamins, minerals list resources:

- https://www.nal.usda.gov/fnic/nutrient-lists-standard-reference-legacy 7.9.21
- https://www.accessdata.fda.gov/scripts/interactivenutri onfactslabel/assets/InteractiveNFL_Vitamins&MineralsC hart_March2020.pdf 7.9.21
- https://www.accessdata.fda.gov/scripts/interactivenutri onfactslabel/factsheets.cfm 7.9.21

CHAPTER 9: SUGAR TRUTHS AND MORE!

1. https://www.ers.usda.gov/topics/crops/sugar-sweeteners/background.aspx 7.15.21
2. American Heart Association - https://www.heart.org/en/healthy-living/healthy-eating/eat-smart/sugar/added-sugars 7.21.20
3. www.nrcs.usda.gov: Why_Eating_a_Little_Slower_Could_Help_You_Lose_W eight (5).pdf 7.19.21
4. https://newsinhealth.nih.gov/special-issues/eating/sweet-stuff / 8.13.20
5. https://www.ncbi.nlm.nih.gov/pmc/articles/PMC4975866 / DiNicolantonio JJ, Berger A. Added sugars drive nutrient and energy deficit in obesity: a new paradigm. Open Heart. 2016 Aug 2;3(2):e000469. doi: 10.1136/openhrt-2016-000469. PMID: 27547437; PMCID: PMC4975866. 8.14.20
6. http://sugarscience.ucsf.edu/ https://sugarscience.ucsf.edu/hidden-in-plain-sight/#.YTZpvI5KiUm 8.9.20

7. https://pubmed.ncbi.nlm.nih.gov/22716101/ Ajibola A, Chamunorwa JP, Erlwanger KH. Nutraceutical values of natural honey and its contribution to human health and wealth. Nutr Metab (Lond). 2012 Jun 20;9:61. doi: 10.1186/1743-7075-9-61. PMID: 22716101; PMCID: PMC3583289. 8.9.20

8. https://fdc.nal.usda.gov/fdc-app.html#/food-details/789126/nutrients / Food Data 8.9.20 honey

9. https://fdc.nal.usda.gov/fdc-app.html#/food-details/789115/nutrients / Food Data 8.9.20 maple syrup

10. https://fdc.nal.usda.gov/fdc-app.html#/food-details/789128/nutrients / Food Data 8.9.20 molasses

11. MedlinePlus, National Library of Medicine: https://medlineplus.gov/fluidandelectrolytebalance.html #:~:text=Electrolytes%20are%20minerals%20in%20your,a cid%2Fbase%20(pH)%20level 8.11.20

12. https://www.cdc.gov/heartdisease/sodium.htm

13. American Heart Association: https://www.heart.org/en/healthy-living/healthy-eating/eat-smart/sodium/how-much-sodium-should-i-eat-per-day 7.21.20 https://www.heart.org/en/healthy-living/healthy-eating/eat-smart/sodium/sodium-sources / 6.5.20

14. https://fdc.nal.usda.gov/index.html / Food Data 8.12.20

15. https://www.accessdata.fda.gov/scripts/interactivenutriti onfactslabel/sodium.cfm / 8.11.20

16. American Heart Association: https://sodiumbreakup.heart.org/21_ingredients_that_me an_sodium_to_watch_on_the_label 8.15.20

17. https://www.cdc.gov/obesity/data/index.html 7.19.21

CHAPTER 10: CLEAN IS SUPREME

1. The Health Effects of Overweight and Obesity, https://www.cdc.gov/healthyweight/effects/index.html 7.24.21

2. https://pubmed.ncbi.nlm.nih.gov/29163542/ Effects of Food Additives on Immune Cells As Contributors to Body Weight Gain and Immune-Mediated Metabolic Dysregulation Paula Neto HA, Ausina P, Gomez LS, Leandro JGB, Zancan P, Sola-Penna M. Effects of Food Additives on Immune Cells As Contributors to Body Weight Gain and Immune-Mediated Metabolic Dysregulation. Front Immunol. 2017;8:1478. Published 2017 Nov 6. doi:10.3389/fimmu.2017.01478 8.30.21

3. https://pubmed.ncbi.nlm.nih.gov/25695045/ Health Safety of Soft Drinks: Contents, Containers, and Microorganisms - Kregiel D. Health safety of soft drinks: contents, containers, and microorganisms. Biomed Res Int. 2015;2015:128697. doi:10.1155/2015/128697 8.30.21

4. https://www.cfsanappsexternal.fda.gov/scripts/fdcc/index.cfm?set=FoodSubstances&id=PHOSPHORICACID 8.18.20

5. https://journals.plos.org/plosone/article?id=10.1371/journal.pone.0000698#abstract0 Citation: Lenoir M, Serre F, Cantin L, Ahmed SH (2007) Intense Sweetness Surpasses Cocaine Reward. PLoS ONE 2(8): e698. https://doi.org/10.1371/journal.pone.0000698 8.8.20

6. https://pubmed.ncbi.nlm.nih.gov/20693348/ Malik VS, Popkin BM, Bray GA, Després JP, Willett WC, Hu FB. Sugar-sweetened beverages and risk of metabolic syndrome and type 2 diabetes: a meta-analysis. Diabetes Care. 2010;33(11):2477-2483. doi:10.2337/dc10-1079 8.30.21

7. https://pubmed.ncbi.nlm.nih.gov/23271574/ Orgel E, Mittelman SD. The links between insulin resistance, diabetes, and cancer. Curr Diab Rep. 2013;13(2):213-222. doi:10.1007/s11892-012-0356-6 8.30.21

8. https://pubmed.ncbi.nlm.nih.gov/29455781/ Purohit V, Mishra S. The truth about artificial sweeteners - Are they good for diabetics?. Indian Heart J. 2018;70(1):197-199. doi:10.1016/j.ihj.2018.01.020 8.21.20

9. https://usrtk.org/sweeteners/aspartame_health_risks/ 8.19.20

10. https://www.fda.gov/food/food-additives-petitions/additional-information-about-high-intensity-sweeteners-permitted-use-food-united-states 8.18.20

11. https://pubmed.ncbi.nlm.nih.gov/11675262/ Tobacman JK. Review of harmful gastrointestinal effects of carrageenan in animal experiments. Environ Health Perspect. 2001;109(10):983-994. doi:10.1289/ehp.01109983 8.18.20

12. https://pubmed.ncbi.nlm.nih.gov/25883986/ 8.18.20 Bhattacharyya S, Feferman L, Unterman T, Tobacman JK. Exposure to common food additive carrageenan alone leads to fasting hyperglycemia and in combination with high fat diet exacerbates glucose intolerance and hyperlipidemia without effect on weight. J Diabetes Res. 2015;2015:513429. doi:10.1155/2015/513429 8.30.21

13. https://pubmed.ncbi.nlm.nih.gov/24761279/ Meredith SE, Juliano LM, Hughes JR, Griffiths RR. Caffeine Use Disorder: A Comprehensive Review and Research Agenda. J Caffeine Res. 2013;3(3):114-130. doi:10.1089/jcr.2013.0016 8.21.20

14. https://www.cdc.gov/niosh/emres/longhourstraining/usingcaffeine.html 8.20.20

15. https://www.fda.gov/consumers/consumer-updates/spilling-beans-how-much-caffeine-too-much 8.21.20

16. https://www.fda.gov/food/food-additives-petitions/questions-and-answers-monosodium-glutamate-msg 8.21.20

17. https://pubmed.ncbi.nlm.nih.gov/29743864/ Niaz K, Zaplatic E, Spoor J. Extensive use of monosodium glutamate: A threat to public health?. EXCLI J. 2018;17:273-278. Published 2018 Mar 19. doi:10.17179/excli2018-1092 8.21.20

18. https://www.fda.gov/food/food-ingredients-packaging/overview-food-ingredients-additives-colors#coloradd 9.7.20

19. https://www.ncbi.nlm.nih.gov/pmc/articles/PMC2957945/Potera C. The artificial food dye blues. Environ Health Perspect. 2010;118(10):A428. doi:10.1289/ehp.118-a428 8.21.20

20. https://www.fda.gov/consumers/consumer-updates/how-safe-are-color-additives 9.7.20

21. https://www.fda.gov/industry/color-additives/color-additives-history 9.7.20

22. https://www.fda.gov/industry/color-additives 9.7.20

23. https://pubmed.ncbi.nlm.nih.gov/32188080/ Karwowska M, Kononiuk A. Nitrates/Nitrites in Food-Risk for Nitrosative Stress and Benefits. Antioxidants (Basel). 2020 Mar 16;9(3):241. doi: 10.3390/antiox9030241. PMID: 32188080; PMCID: PMC7139399. 10.12.21

24. https://pubs.niaaa.nih.gov/publications/aa22.htm Alcohol Alert 7.24.21

25. https://www.cdc.gov/alcohol/pdfs/alcoholyourhealth.pdf 7.24.21

26. https://www.nhtsa.gov/risky-driving/drunk-driving 8.24.20

27. https://www.ttb.gov/other/regulations#alcohol 8.25.20

28. http://npic.orst.edu/factsheets/glyphogen.html 8.29.20

29. https://usrtk.org/pesticides/glyphosate-health-concerns/ 8.29.20

30. https://www.usda.gov/our-agency/about-usda 8.29.21

31. https://www.nass.usda.gov/Publications/Highlights/2020 /census-organics.pdf 7.24.21

32. https://www.ams.usda.gov/about-ams/programs-offices/national-organic-program 7.24.21

33. https://ota.com/advocacy/organic-standards/national-list-allowed-and-prohibited-substances 8.21.20

34. https://www.ams.usda.gov/grades-standards/organic-standards 8.21.20

35. https://www.fda.gov/food/food-labeling-nutrition/use-term-natural-food-labeling 7.24.21

36. https://www.fsis.usda.gov/food-safety/safe-food-handling-and-preparation/poultry/poultry-label-says-fresh 7.24.21

37. https://www.ams.usda.gov/publications/qa-shell-eggs 9.7.20

38. https://www.fisheries.noaa.gov/insight/understanding-sustainable-seafood 9.1.20

39. https://www.nal.usda.gov/afsic/organic-aquaculture 9.1.20

40. https://www.fishwatch.gov/sustainable-seafood/the-global-picture 9.1.20

41. https://usrtk.org/pesticides/glyphosate-health-concerns

42. https://pubmed.ncbi.nlm.nih.gov/24426015/ Bawa AS, Anilakumar KR. Genetically modified foods: safety, risks and public concerns-a review. J Food Sci Technol.

2013;50(6):1035-1046. doi:10.1007/s13197-012-0899-1
8.21.20

43. https://www.fda.gov/food/agricultural-
biotechnology/gmo-crops-animal-food-and-beyond
7.24.21

44. https://www.fda.gov/food/food-labeling-nutrition/food-
allergies

45. https://www.fda.gov/food/food-labeling-
nutrition/changes-nutrition-facts-label 9.2.20

46. https://pubmed.ncbi.nlm.nih.gov/22481896/ de Lourdes
Samaniego-Vaesken M, Alonso-Aperte E, Varela-
Moreiras G. Vitamin food fortification today. Food Nutr
Res. 2012;56:10.3402/fnr.v56i0.5459.
doi:10.3402/fnr.v56i0.5459   9.2.20

CHAPTER 11: HOW YOUR BODY COMMUNICATES TO YOU

1. https://pubmed.ncbi.nlm.nih.gov/32572435/ Li JH, Duan
R, Li L, Wood JD, Wang XY, Shu Y, Wang GD. [Unique
characteristics of "the second brain" - The enteric nervous
system]. Sheng Li Xue Bao. 2020 Jun 25;72(3):382-390.
Chinese. PMID: 32572435.Li JH, Duan R, Li L, et al. Sheng
Li Xue Bao. 2020;72(3):382-390. 7.26.21

2. https://pubmed.ncbi.nlm.nih.gov/29427583 Sylvia KE,
Demas GE. A gut feeling: Microbiome-brain-immune
interactions modulate social and affective behaviors.
Horm Behav. 2018 Mar;99:41-49. doi:
10.1016/j.yhbeh.2018.02.001. Epub 2018 Feb 20. PMID:
29427583; PMCID: PMC5880698   7.26.21

3. https://www.sleepfoundation.org/articles/what-
circadian-rhythm 3.29.20

CHAPTER 13: HEALING SLEEP

1. https://www.cdc.gov/sleep/about_sleep/chronic_disease. htl 4.17.20

2. https://www.nrcs.usda.gov/wps/portal/nrcs/detail/ks/peo ple/employees/?cid=nrcs142p2_033304 8.3.21

3. https://www.nrcs.usda.gov/wps/portal/nrcs/detail/ks/peo ple/employees/?cid=nrcs142p2_033304 myths about sleep 7.18.21

4. https://pubmed.ncbi.nlm.nih.gov/22038945/ Ludy MJ, Moore GE, Mattes RD. The effects of capsaicin and capsiate on energy balance: critical review and meta-analyses of studies in humans. Chem Senses. 2012 Feb;37(2):103-21. doi: 10.1093/chemse/bjr100. Epub 2011 Oct 29. PMID: 22038945; PMCID: PMC3257466. 8.2.21

5. https://www.ninds.nih.gov/Disorders/Patient-Caregiver-Education/Understanding-Sleep 8.2.21

6. https://www.sleepfoundation.org/sleep-deprivation 8.2.21

7. https://www.sleepfoundation.org/circadian-rhythm 8.2.21

8. https://pubmed.ncbi.nlm.nih.gov/32230944/ Binks H, E Vincent G, Gupta C, Irwin C, Khalesi S. Effects of Diet on Sleep: A Narrative Review. Nutrients. 2020 Mar 27;12(4):936. doi: 10.3390/nu12040936. PMID: 32230944; PMCID: PMC7230229. 8.3.21

9. https://pubmed.ncbi.nlm.nih.gov/28387721/ Meng X, Li Y, Li S, Zhou Y, Gan RY, Xu DP, Li HB. Dietary Sources and Bioactivities of Melatonin. Nutrients. 2017 Apr 7;9(4):367. doi: 10.3390/nu9040367. PMID: 28387721; PMCID: PMC5409706. 8.2.21

CHAPTER 14: MINDFULNESS

1. https://pubmed.ncbi.nlm.nih.gov/29996822/ Tao L, Yang K, Huang F, Liu X, Li X, Luo Y, Wu L, Guo X. Association between self-reported eating speed and metabolic syndrome in a Beijing adult population: a cross-sectional study. BMC Public Health. 2018 Jul 11;18(1):855. doi: 10.1186/s12889-018-5784-z. PMID: 29996822; PMCID: PMC6042428. 8.6.21

CHAPTER 16: GET SMART, GET READY, GO!

Permission granted to use Zig Ziglar quote (www.ziglar.com) 7.15.20